ADVANCE PRAISE FOR
POSITIVE SLEEP
(FIRST ~~EDITION~~

"This book is a roadmap for an,
a personal and engaging way, Giles offers insights and practical steps that
will not only improve your sleep but also improve your life. A must-read."

JAMES BURSTALL

Founder and Group CEO, Argonon, bestselling author,
The Flexible Method: Prepare to Prosper in the Next Global Crisis

"Giles Watkins has taken a subject dear to almost everyone's hearts and –
in simple, accessible and very personal terms – laid it out for us all to see.
The result is a readable and practical book stacked full of stories and
examples that constitutes a courageous call to personal action."

MIKE CARSON

Partner, McKinsey & Company, Founding Partner, Aberkyn, author,
The Manager – Inside the Minds of Football's Leaders

"Positive Sleep *is one of the most practical books on sleep I have read.
Giles takes an approach that includes the bigger picture while deep diving
into details. The pragmatic suggestions interwoven with personal anecdotes
and scientific studies make for compelling reading.*"

CELYNN MORIN

Workplace wellbeing whisperer

"*Positive Sleep combines the latest neuroscience and Giles's personal experiences to explain why sleep is so important to healthy living. Giles explores the impact that sleep deprivation has on all of us. More importantly, he also explores how sleep in the right quantity and quality can boost the positive leadership behaviours so needed in corporations today.*

"*This book promises no magic wand but offers lots of practical advice for individuals and organizations to promote good sleep patterns, a healthier lifestyle and better work environment. This is a must-read for anyone in a global corporation dealing with late night conference calls, early morning international flights and the demands of being 'on call' 24/7. It's a valuable guide for anyone who has spent the night tossing and turning and suffered the next day as a result.*"

ROMY MURRAY

Non-Executive Director (international financial services) and executive coach

"*A candid and practical book from a reformed corporate workaholic that will inspire you to take a more holistic view of your life, your health and the steps you can take to harness your most vital health resource – sleep.*"

JO MACSWEEN

Leadership coach and peer group facilitator

"*Sleep deprivation is an internationally recognized means of torture, yet millions of us deliberately do it to ourselves, and millions more don't take it seriously enough. This book contains excellent practical tips on how to make good sleep the centrepiece of our approach to better health and wellbeing.*"

P.B. SUBBIAH

HR Director

"Giles Watkins intertwines the compelling narrative of his own struggles with sleep with academic research and other sleep literature to provide a convincing argument for the importance of sleep for our work, our relationships and our wellbeing. Giles outlines in clear, fluent writing the steps involved in taking an effective holistic approach to help us get the positive sleep we need and demonstrates why all of us – organizations, institutions and individuals – need to wake up to the essential role sleep plays in our lives. Positive Sleep is the book you should take to bed with you!"

JACK PINTER
Founder, Square One Partnership, facilitator, playwright and saxophonist

"Giles Watkins's Positive Sleep is an honest and frank account of the challenges that millions face about getting 'good' sleep and the multiple factors that affect our sleep from both a personal and professional level. If there was one thing that could positively benefit organizations and individuals in terms of resilience, it would be better sleep! From both a physiological and psychological perspective we are built to need sleep; this is something we can't cheat or evolve beyond. The data and science is clear – on a basic level, brain, immune and mental health are intrinsically linked to sleep. Positive Sleep provides a valuable insight into the tools, strategies and mindset needed to support better sleep, as there is no magic bullet. An informative and insightful read."

KATE FISMER BSC
MRN, lead consultant, Centre for Resilience at the University of Westminster and Director, Revolution Resilience

"Positive Sleep is an important book tackling a crucial issue. Giles combines hard-won personal experience with rigorous research in this gem of a read. Enlightening and instructive."

NIGEL MARSH
Author, Fat, Forty and Fired, and creator and host, The Five Of My Life

"Giles's personal journey is an inspiration to all. His honest account of looking for deeper insights reads like a novel. It makes it easy to relate to and puts it well above many of the 'how to' books in this genre. If you ever thought of maximizing your productivity by cutting on sleep, this book will give you some food for thought. Its holistic approach is a pillar for individual wellbeing and the sustainable relationships these times call for."

TONY VERBRAEKEN

HR Executive Vice President, Shell

"Poor sleep quality is dangerous. It generates stress, undermines performance and erodes our health and wellbeing. Learning to sleep well needs our urgent attention. Giles Watkins offers us insights which are not only practical and well researched, but also engaging and accessible. I commend his work; it could change your life for the better."

NARENDRA LALJANI

Management educator, strategy consultant, CEO coach and board member

"I found it to be a very enlightening and personal account with practical advice, supported by solid research and science, to combat one of the modern plagues in our society that is interested in 'what we do' rather than 'who we are'. Here is a successful jet set executive getting thrown into the jaws of busy-ness (rather than business), destroying health, family and morality to fulfil the diktat of what success should look like ... and it provides the data to support (or rationalize) daily naps!"

LOIC SADOULET

Affiliate Professor of Economics, INSEAD

Published by
LID Publishing
An imprint of LID Business Media Ltd.
LABS House, 15-19 Bloomsbury Way,
London, WC1A 2TH, UK

info@lidpublishing.com
www.lidpublishing.com

A member of:
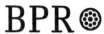
businesspublishersroundtable.com

Printed and bound in Great Britain by Halstan Ltd

ISBN: 978-1-915951-32-8
ISBN: 978-1-915951-33-5 (ebook)

Cover and page design: Caroline Li
Illustrated by Alistair Bullen and Dan White

THE POSITIVE SLEEP BOOK

A HOLISTIC APPROACH TO RESOLVE
SLEEP ISSUES AND TRANSFORM YOUR LIFE

GILES WATKINS

MADRID | MEXICO CITY | LONDON
BUENOS AIRES | BOGOTA | SHANGHAI

FOR OTHER TITLES
IN THE SERIES ...

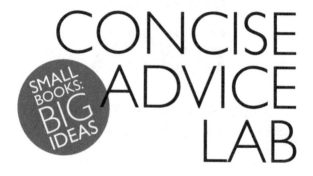

CONCISE
ADVICE
LAB

SMALL BOOKS: BIG IDEAS

CLEVER CONTENT, DYNAMIC IDEAS, PRACTICAL
SOLUTIONS AND ENGAGING VISUALS –
A CATALYST TO INSPIRE NEW WAYS OF THINKING
AND PROBLEM-SOLVING IN A COMPLEX WORLD

www.lidpublishing.com/product-category/concise-advice-series

CONTENTS

For Elliott – who always makes getting
a decent night's sleep worthwhile

And Philip Goldman (1956–2023)
Friend and mentor

ACKNOWLEDGMENTS

I would like to thank Elizabeth Florent-Treacy, whose wisdom was the catalyst to my choosing both sleep and an auto-ethnographical approach for my original thesis, written as part of my Executive Master's programme in Coaching and Consulting for Change at INSEAD in Singapore. This would prove to be a life-changing decision for me, for which I am truly grateful.

Also thanks to my thesis editor, Kah Ying Choo, for her skill, authenticity and professionalism over the period of more than two years that we worked together. Without you, this thesis would never have been completed.

To my many teachers and peers from Wave 16 of the INSEAD programme in Singapore who walked with me along the journey. Thank you all for providing the key inspiration for my transformation.

Also to Paul Forman and Simon Youngs at Coats Group plc, whose sponsorship of my enthusiasm to undertake the Master's programme enabled me to do so.

I would never have written a book without the encouragement of Ben Renshaw, who was an early 'coach' of mine. We first worked together in 1999, and meeting Ben for a cuppa (no caffeine, of course!) in July 2018 led to the writing and publishing of *Positive Sleep*.

To all at LID – you more than justified Ben's recommendation! I must single out LID's Head of Publishing at the time for particular praise. Always both thoughtful and timely in her responses, Sara Taheri really pulled *Positive Sleep* together from the strands that I've written.

My illustrator Alistair Bullen, founder of ABA, has brought each part of the book to life with his drawings. Thanks Al for hatching the idea to work on this in the first place during a washed-out day at Lord's Cricket Ground and for honouring your promise as always. And thanks to Dan White for the new additions to *The Positive Sleep Book*.

Ashok Ferrey, Sri Lanka's leading English language author still resident in the country, was constantly telling me I had a voice and should write something when I lived and worked in Colombo between 2010 and 2014. Thanks Ashok – you were right.

The Next Business School in Colombo, Sri Lanka gave me my first paid talk on Sleep. Thanks to Kumudu Abeyawardane and her team for their faith in me.

The Peer Group Advisory Board of SME CEOs that I run through Vistage have not only let me practise some of my theories on them, but have also given me feedback that's been incredibly perceptive and useful. Thanks to Claire Bodanis, Paul Turnbull, Quentin Crowe,

Matt Gray, Tao Xing, Luke Redman and most especially Ashley Hayward, who also lent me the exceptional 'Think' room at Workplace House, Kinnarps UK's London Showroom, to write in.

Claire Bodanis also introduced me to fellow Dark Angels John Simmons and Martin Lee who shared their wisdom on how to write. Please don't blame them for the results! Their tips certainly helped me to enjoy the process more.

My colleagues within the Aberkyn (a wholly owned member of the McKinsey family of firms), who have so often generated great insights to support me on the writing path. In particular, Jack Pinter, Neil Pearse, Mike Carson and Maggie Elis have been a constant source of encouragement to me in the latter stages of writing.

Andy Wolfe and Mark Albas of Arcadia Consulting have been key in helping me improve my executive presence to communicate the key insights from this book face to face. I'm most grateful to you both in helping me get my message out there to assist others in this way. Thanks to Kim Raine – you raised my awareness of the connection between diet, exercise and sleep and inspired me to kick my coffee addiction.

A number of people who have read the book have been generous with their endorsements: Neil Mullarkey, Nigel Marsh, James Burstall, Celynn Morin, Ben Renshaw, Nikki Owen, Els van der Helm, Jan Lloyd, Mark Albas, Ashok Ferrey, Romy Murray, Mike Carson, Lena Parker, Jo Macsween, Jack Pinter, Jeremy Snape, Kate Fismer, Marjorie Brown, P.B. Subbiah, Tony Verbraeken, Narendra Laljani, Loic Sadoulet, Nikki Gerling and Tanya Kabalin. Sincere thanks to you all.

Particular thanks to Steve Pickering and all at Sussex Beds.

To my Mum and Dad – for many things, including inspiring a love of napping! And to Nick, Jess and Sue for their love and support along life's journey.

To Sophie, who endured the bad bits and inspired the writing of this, thanks for your love and patience.

To Elliott – I trust that you will learn from your dad's mistakes and value a good night's sleep as the foundation of health and as a cornerstone of success.

Most specifically for the second edition, I'd like to acknowledge the constant support and encouragement of Rob Hingston and his team at Origin Workspace, where most of the new material was written.

My alma mater, the University of Bristol, has been a great source of inspiration and wisdom in recent years. I'd like to acknowledge the ongoing support of Professor Matt Jones and his colleagues in the Department of Neuroscience, plus students at the Centre for Innovation and Entrepreneurship.

And to LMS and FMS – you know who you are.

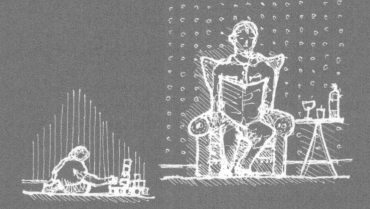

PART ONE

INTRODUCTION

CHAPTER 1:
BACKGROUND

The issue of 'sleep difficulties' is an oft-neglected topic that affects many people today. Having struggled myself with sleep problems for over a decade and, ultimately, having identified potentially effective solutions, I am constantly being asked how sleep challenges can be overcome. Anywhere, from presentations I run for groups about sleep to informal chats at the bus stop, people love to talk about sleep! Whatever the sleep challenges stem from – work pressures, relationship issues, becoming a parent and so on – lack of sleep can easily dominate your life, as it did mine. So, although numerous institutions such as the Harvard Medical School have promoted sleep as a foundational pillar of health together with diet and exercise, literally hundreds of millions of people are suffering the health effects of lack of sleep – physical, mental and emotional.

To many it feels like our days and nights are under attack. In post-industrial societies it seems that many regard sleep as simply time wasted which could be put to other, more worthwhile uses. In *The Sleep Revolution*, Arianna Huffington[1] illustrates the depth of the problem when she quotes the US Surgeon General Dr Vivek Murthy. "Health is deeply intertwined with culture: what we eat, how active we are, how much we sleep," said Dr Murthy. "When I was training in medicine for example, there was a culture that strong people didn't need sleep ... It is not helpful to have a culture that supports unhealthy practices like that." So, if the medical profession is not truly behind promoting healthy sleep in society and being a role model for this behaviour, many of the rest of us follow.

One of the main reasons for this is our increasing focus on work, partially derived from attainment at work and the wealth that can accumulate from it. Material riches and the associated status that derives from this is seen as a hallmark of success. And now that so many of us can carry our work around with us on portable devices the pressure to work is always there.

Take the example of sleep deprivation – for a short or prolonged period of time – now an issue of 'epidemic proportions' among professionals according to Theo Compernolle in his book *Brain Chains*.[2] Not only do the effects of sleep deprivation undermine an individual's ability to engage in important forms of leadership behaviours, in the long run they may also adversely affect the financial performance of their organizations.[3] In a survey of 2,500 managers in five countries (the UK, US, Netherlands, Japan and Germany) it was revealed that the average amount of sleep of a manager was lower than the 'recommended number of hours' by 19%. Moreover, as a result of insufficient sleep, levels of concentration, patience and enthusiasm were adversely affected in half of those surveyed.[4]

The good news is that although sleep behaviours are an intensely personal issue, employers are finally 'waking up' to their responsibility for contributing to this problem. In an increasingly hyperconnected world, many companies now expect their employees to

Health is deeply intertwined with culture: what we eat, how active we are, how much we sleep.

Dr Vivek Murthy,
US Surgeon General

be on call and to answer emails 24/7. The existence of a sleep problem among executives is further borne out by McKinsey's survey of 196 business leaders. Overall, 66% and 55% reported that they were generally dissatisfied with their sleep quantity and sleep quality, respectively. Over 80% of the respondents reported that the education provided by their organizations regarding the significance of sleep had been limited. Furthermore, 47% of the leaders stated that they were expected to be available via emails and phone calls for unreasonably long periods. Yet 46% of respondents believed that a lack of sleep exerted little impact on their leadership performance, thus highlighting how much individuals and organizations are in denial about their struggle with sleep issues.[5]

The complacency of employers and employees reflects a lack of knowledge and awareness of the importance of sleep. Neuroscientists have found that, although other brain areas can cope relatively well with insufficient sleep, the prefrontal cortex that is responsible for executive functioning, including all the higher-order cognitive processes such as planning and executing plans, is greatly affected.[6, 7] Diverse research studies on the effects of sleep deprivation on executive functioning to specific leadership behaviours[8] showed that sleep deprivation can adversely affect behaviours that are key to good leadership: the ability to stay focused on results, solve problems, evaluate the viability of different perspectives and help others. Essentially, an individual's struggle with sleep difficulties and sleep deprivation should be of critical concern to the organization they work for and the 'family' they live within, as well as to them as individuals.

Individuals, organizations and society as a whole cannot continue to turn a blind eye to the existence of this issue, nor ignore their roles in exaccrbating the problem. And part of the challenge in addressing this is that the study of sleep is still relatively new in comparison to other branches of science, having largely developed over the last 100 years.

"That's all very interesting!" I hear you cry. "However, what is sleep? Why does it matter? And how can I improve my sleep tonight?!"

Well, that's precisely what I will aim to address in this book. Much of this is based on my own experience in addressing my own sleep issues. However, a word of warning in advance! Ultimately, the solution for my sleep challenges did not lie in specialized assistance or tools related to the area of sleep. Nor did it come from the land of quick fixes, apps or 'off the shelf' solutions. Far more beneficial to me has been the adoption of a more holistic approach – changing my lifestyle and habits including those relating to diet and fitness, including mindset and attitude towards work and relationships. In this way I not only eliminated my sleep issues but also transformed my life. So, while I offer tips that can be immediately implemented to help you sleep better, the most sustainable approach will take a little longer to formulate. However, the effort required for good sleep is worthwhile since sleep makes up for a third of our life, which then provides the platform to both nourish and optimize the other two thirds!

CHAPTER 2:
MY INTEREST IN
THIS TOPIC

My struggle with sleep difficulties began more than two decades ago in 2002, being a slight inconvenience at the start of the problem and escalating to adversely affecting every sphere of my life. During this period, I made a few unsuccessful attempts to address the problem, either by seeking specialized professional assistance or using DIY approaches. With the benefit of hindsight, it was evident that they were doomed to fail because I had adopted a half-hearted approach. Moreover, each of these approaches did not delve into the heart of the problem or consider the complex interaction of multiple factors.

In 2014, as part of my Executive Master's at the INSEAD Business School in Singapore, I was asked to reflect on potential topics for a thesis. As lack of quality and quantity of sleep had now become a chronic and debilitating condition for me, this assignment struck me as the perfect opportunity to address something that was ruining my quality of life, my marriage and, no doubt, my long-term health too. In my endeavour to find a solution for my condition, I was also motivated by the possibility that my thesis could also generate answers for others in similar straits. This was just as well because

I did not quite bargain for the pain I'd endure in the process, both physically (through detoxes, for example) and emotionally (as the thesis required an in-depth reflection on my feelings and fears which at times lay outside my conscious awareness).

With this book my aim is to share what I've learned from my research and help you understand why sleep matters and to identify effective treatments and strategies to empower you to sleep better (whatever that means for you). Through the exploration of my own sleep issues and eliciting my own insights, it is my hope that my findings will be helpful for others in similar circumstances.

CHAPTER 3:
SLEEP AND COVID-19

It would be a delightful – some would say typically British – understatement to say that the world has changed significantly since *Positive Sleep: A Holistic Approach to Resolve Sleep Issues and Transform Your Life* was first published in 2019. The impact of COVID-19 was felt pretty much globally and many people's sleep suffered as a result. Hence the big shifts in how we live, plus where, when, and indeed why we work is part of the reason for this second edition. These shifts in behaviour are starting to show new patterns for many, whilst being nowhere near equilibrium as employees and employers attempt to reconcile conflicting wishes.

Add to these recent developments in Artificial Intelligence and Quantum Computing over the last few years, plus wars in Ukraine and the Middle East, and it's easy to feel that the 'new normal' is a state of disequilibrium.

Like most of us, I had to adapt my work during COVID-19, spreading the Positive Sleep message from in-person workshops and keynotes to online events via Zoom, Microsoft Teams and the like. One upside was that I took this opportunity to run online polls before – or at the start of – these sessions and focused the questions on exploring the typical quantity of sleep the delegates were getting in a 24-hour period, and if that had changed since COVID-19 lockdowns began. The responses, from an audience working for clients as diverse as Google Singapore, Santander UK Commercial and the pizza oven makers Ooni, were surprisingly uniform. Typically, about two thirds of the respondents reported a change in the amount of sleep they were currently enjoying. And, of those two thirds, approximately two thirds thought they were sleeping less, whereas one third said they slept longer.

COVID-19 LOCKDOWNS AFFECT ON SLEEP QUALITY

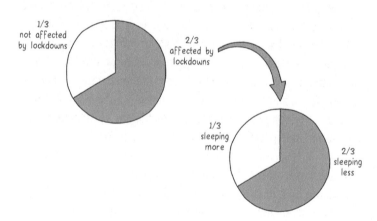

1/3
not affected
by lockdowns

2/3
affected by
lockdowns

1/3
sleeping
more

2/3
sleeping
less

SOURCE: Online polls conducted by the author with employees of Google Singapore, Santander UK Commercial and Ooni (2020/21)

So how did these small-scale snapshots (of circa 25) match the evolving picture of larger studies? Well, in the earliest days of COVID-19, two studies were published that showed a divergent picture. One study by Fitbit in April 2020[1] was based on data gathered in the second half of March in both the US and Europe. In both, an average increase in the time slept was noted. In the US, the Fitbit findings noted a state-by-state picture ranging from an increase in sleep of 25 minutes per night to a slight reduction of circa five minutes. This seemed to chime reasonably well with the European data gathered in the cities of London, Zürich, Barcelona, Madrid, Milan and Paris, showing that Fitbit users were sleeping an average of 13 to 25 minutes more per night.

However, The Sleep Council in the UK (along with its partners the Sleep Charity and Sleep Station) published a study at the end of April 2020 showing a different trend in the UK.[2] Here, it appears that about half the respondents found it harder to fall asleep and three quarters admitted that a lack of sleep was interfering with their ability to function during the day. Results from Italy indicated something similar. One plausible explanation is that this survey was taken about a month later than the Fitbit findings.

As I write this, several years after the arrival of COVID-19, there is a growing body of evidence of the pandemic being the cause of both short- and long-term sleep issues.[3] One example is The Sleep Foundation's research, which showed that "although sleep problems are not frequently listed amongst the key symptoms, an analysis across countries found that around 52% of people with COVID-19 have sleep disruptions." And not sleeping well is likely to slow your recovery, as it plays such an important role in repair, recuperation and getting your immune system back on track.[4]

Such affects led to the coining of the term Coronasomnia, a colloquial rather than official or medical term, describing the wider implications for sleep of the pandemic beyond those who suffered from the SARS-COVID-2 coronavirus. Hence the term Coronasomnia includes the following:

Disrupted routines – many different work and domestic pressures throw our typical daily schedules into disarray, affecting our internal clock (or circadian rhythm), creating a higher risk of sleep disruptions.

Isolation – many people were more isolated than usual in the pandemic, which often led to a reduction in emotional health and sleep. And in many cases, they have never recovered these pre-pandemic patterns.

Stress – the uncertainty generated by the pandemic heightened stress for many, leading to sleep loss.

Pandemic fatigue – supposedly especially common in people who follow the news closely. Perhaps watching the 10 o'clock news every night is bad for your health?!

Caregiving roles – the pandemic appears to have been especially disruptive and stressful for those with school-aged children for multiple reasons, linked again to loss of routine, and home schooling.

Mental health challenges – well documented anecdotally, with a survey from the Lancet showing increased levels across multiple countries.[5]

Undiagnosed sleep disorders – such as obstructive sleep apnea (OSA). This could have multiple causes, including restricted access to certain care facilities, such as sleep labs and other medical facilities during/post-pandemic.

Reduced medical care – linked to the point above. Many people have avoided seeking non-urgent medical care, and hence some issues are going untreated despite the resulting loss of sleep.

The Sleep Foundation's findings on what is now commonly known as Long Covid suggests that >30% of sufferers struggle with sleep.[6] In addition to chronic insomnia and mental health challenges, some of the pain and shortness of breath associated with COVID can linger for weeks and months afterwards. Changes in sleep architecture have been observed, less deep sleep in particular, and delayed circadian rhythm has also been reported.

Having already discussed some of the shifts that have occurred with sleep patterns, I will look at some of the opportunities and threats from technological advances that could affect our sleep in the penultimate chapters.

CHAPTER 4: LAUNCHING AN ACTIVE QUEST FOR ANSWERS

I was blessed to have the opportunity of a reorganization at work that prompted me to return to the UK about ten years ago, and also inspired a reassessment of my health as I was approaching 50. Moving from a less developed country where the medical services were simply not equipped to address sleep issues, and coming back home to live in the UK also provided me with an opportunity to seek out professional assistance with my sleep. I was now studying the topic of sleep and gathering data on my own sleep through an electronic device, so I'd become pretty good at defining the problem – all I needed now were some solutions.

At the start of my investigative journey, my strategies centred on using specialized devices and specialists targeted at addressing sleep issues. Initially, I purchased a Jawbone device which I wore on my wrist for a period of nine months in order to monitor my sleeping hours. Then, in November 2014, I went to my GP to get a referral letter for a private sleep consultation. My GP prescribed melatonin and trazodone to help me to sleep, dismissing my sleep issues as being not too bad compared to his. I chose not to get the prescription filled, as I was not looking for a pharmaceutical solution. I was utterly disappointed by this consultation: after struggling with my sleep issues for more than a decade and finally seeking help, I felt the medical professional had failed to take my sleep issue seriously.

Armed with the GP's referral letter, I subsequently went through two specialized sleep consultations and an examination, which yielded two treatment interventions. First, Professor Adrian Williams, Professor of Sleep Medicine at King's College in London, diagnosed me with moderate obstructive sleep apnoea (OSA) and recommended the fitting of a continuous positive airway pressure (CPAP) device. The CPAP is a small pump that delivers a continuous supply of compressed air through a mask that prevents the throat from closing – it is this closing of the throat that produces the snoring noise and gasping. He also proposed cognitive behavioural therapy (CBT). I was reluctant to proceed with CBT, as I suspected that the root causes were my marital and work issues and I was not convinced that CBT would help me fix them. Of course, this rationale could be masking my underlying fears about my marriage and concern that I would never sleep well again. I also learned that my British private health insurance did not cover my consultation; it seemed that the British medical establishment did not consider sleep issues to be a medical problem at that time.

In fairness, I should note that CBT-I has become much more widely available since then. It is an insomnia-specific psychological therapy for adults with insomnia, which has been proven to work effectively in a whole range of research trials. However, I have not tried it myself and am not in a position to evaluate its efficacy beyong what I've read.

So, after all that, where was I? With a greater understanding of my OSA, my foray into sleep-oriented solutions had only confirmed the existence of my sleep problems. According to the Jawbone device, I was averaging 5–6 hours of sleep per night. However, this figure masked the erratic nature of my actual sleeping patterns. Typically, I slept for 3–4 hours per night about twice a week, waking up between 1am and 3am and being unable to get back to sleep. Then I made up for it by sleeping longer on other nights. I continued to be tired at work, napping whenever I could during the weekends.

Due to my discouraging experiences with medical providers, I was spurred to seek out solutions elsewhere. My breakthrough came in early March 2015 when I read *The Sleep Book* by Dr Guy Meadows.[1] This book affirmed my growing perception that mindfulness might hold the key to improved sleep: sleeping better was all about 'being' rather than 'doing'. I had probably become more open to this statement due to my years of excessive working and the toll this had taken. My introspectiveness was also bolstered by my exposure to the Master's programme I was studying at INSEAD. This taught me the concept of 'Night Vision,' which encouraged me to "see into the dark corners of [my] awareness where essences of the issue might be lurking".[2] Thus, I felt that engaging in more reflection would enable me to find the answer to my sleep problem, rather than doing more stuff to fix it.

I was now using a range of mindfulness techniques to get back to sleep, the most effective of these being the one I call 'Body Scanning', also known as 'Noticing Sensations and Urges'. This involves moving your awareness into your body and noticing emotions, physical sensations or urges that exist there. You start with your toes and slowly scan up through your whole body until you reach the top of your head, stopping for 10–30 seconds on each area and bringing your awareness to it. Take this opportunity to really notice whatever you feel here and then thank that part of the body for what it contributes to your overall functioning on a daily basis.

This technique proved very effective in helping me get back to sleep in the middle of the night by allowing me to tune in to my body, one area at a time. So, although I still woke up at 3am, I often got at least another hour of sleep between 3am and 5.30am. And on the rare occasions I could not get back to sleep, I found myself seduced into a trancelike state which was incredibly restful and so much more pleasant than simply tossing and turning and not being able to get back to sleep. By getting about seven hours of sleep on a regular basis, I no longer needed to nap during the day, which allowed me to play soccer and cricket with my son Elliott in the park on weekends. This change in my life thus felt like the beginnings of a 'virtuous circle': having more energy to seek out other ways to change my situation enabled me to overcome my own resistance to change and to transform.

Building upon this success, I asked around for someone I could work with to help me improve my diet and exercise, figuring that these were the other two pillars of health, along with sleep. I started working with Kim Raine, a fitness and diet coach, in July 2015, who initiated me on a new diet and fitness regimen to support and sustain my improving sleep habit. I committed myself to a month of 'eating clean' – no coffee and bread, minimal alcohol, natural carbohydrates only (e.g. brown rice and sweet potatoes) – and high-protein foods after exercise. My exercise activity began with regular walks for the first month, followed by some routine exercises to strengthen my core muscles. Then I alternated between running (especially interval training) with gym work and spinning classes up to six times per week. Over a six-month period, I lost 5kg on this regime and improved my fitness levels. I was able to play in the park with Elliott for far longer periods of time than before.

In addition, Kim also provided me with a number of sleep meditations that I could listen to whenever I needed them to fall asleep. I also changed my evening routine with her encouragement. At around 9.30pm, I would take a warm detoxifying bath with Epsom salts each night for about 20 minutes. After that, Sophie, my wife, and I would watch one or two episodes of a mini-series on Netflix until 10.30 or even 11pm. I discovered that I had no problem staying awake to watch them. By staying up later in the evening, I was now waking up at 5.30 or 6am regularly, occasionally even after 7am, having either slept right through the night or having got up just the once to visit the bathroom.

Finally, I added a new morning routine – a daily meditation that involved sitting up straight or in a half-lotus position, while reflecting on passing thoughts and letting them go without fixating on any one train of thought. Overall, the meditation routine has helped me to be more in the moment and contribute to my general wellbeing. I'd tried meditation before and always felt that I was not doing it properly for some reason. Ultimately, I came to realize that there was really no right or wrong answer when it came to the practice of meditation, and that's exactly what it was – a practice! So, I started with less than five minutes a day and built up. I now typically enjoy 15–20 minutes of practice each morning, using some meditation beads – called a 'mala' by yoga practitioners – so that I keep in a rhythm of breathing and have an approximate idea how long it will take.

Thanks to Kim's interventions and meditations, I progressed in improving my sleeping habits and in significantly reducing my snoring issue. In January 2016, the doctor and I agreed to postpone the use of the CPAP device.

Although I had tried to make lifestyle changes in the past, my earlier endeavours to adopt a healthier lifestyle were often misguided because I had no proper professional guidance. But what is of note is that my own personal investment of around £2,000 in sleep expertise did not yield a solution. The ultimate solution came in the form of sustained lifestyle changes and simple techniques that brought greater calm into my life. Changing to a 'human being' from a 'human doing' brought clear benefits to me which, in turn, improved my sleep.

Therefore, in reviewing the trajectory of my sleep patterns over the previous decades, I could see that my sleep difficulties were years in the making. While I had been able to keep up with this hectic lifestyle during my early years, I was no longer able to do so once I reached the midlife phase. And perhaps, most significantly, I had also made a major change in my life by quitting my corporate job in December 2015. Leading businesses involving hundreds of employees and turnovers of hundreds of millions of dollars in countries and cultures that were not my own, and pursuing an accompanying hectic social life, no longer felt like the authentic me. My transformation from being reactive to creative, which motivated me to strive to be the best version of me, was probably instrumental in enabling me to stick to Kim's disciplined regimen. What is also true is that 'clean eating' is truly a virtuous circle. Once I started this and stuck with it my physical cravings for certain types of food subsided. Here it was the social pressures (especially with regards to alcohol) that enticed me back to a less clean diet rather than my own cravings.

And without question, the reflection and 'unpeeling of the onion' that I had engaged in during the Master's programme influenced my approach to life and gave me the courage and energy to address my sleep difficulties. Chronicling my sleep history for the thesis helped me to get to the bottom of my sleep issues.

On a deeper level, I recognized that my tendency to suppress my emotions and my hectic work-oriented lifestyle had adversely affected the quality of my life. My sleep difficulties were symptomatic of many underlying things that I needed to change. In resolving them and improving the quality of my sleep, I have gained a new lease of life and acquired new insights that could be helpful in addressing the sleep difficulties of other professionals like myself.

My sleep difficulties were symptomatic of many underlying things that I needed to change.

CHAPTER 5: TRIGGERING EVENT WITH LINGERING AFTERMATH

If I was to pinpoint the start of my debilitating sleep difficulties, it would be the episode involving my organization of a face-to-face offsite programme for my global team in April 2002. This was when I was 37. From that episode onwards, I began to experience sleep difficulties that affected my work day. This sleep pattern would plague me for more than a decade ...

About 90 minutes into day one of the four-day programme, our then boss, C.C., arrived to make an announcement: the team would be dissolved before Christmas because the company was undergoing a major reorganization. All team members would have to find new positions or be made redundant. After that, no one could concentrate on the agenda, so within an hour the boss ripped up the plan and we spent the rest of the day having various discussions to get into the best possible frame of mind to cope with what was to come. Although I slept soundly after going to bed around midnight, I awoke before 5am the next day – an hour earlier than usual. At the time, I did not think that there was anything untoward about my waking up an hour earlier. I had risen early to send an email summary of the key takeaways of the previous evening's session at C.C.'s request.

In retrospect, I recognized that I had suppressed my true feelings for both professional and personal reasons. As the organizer of the meeting, I felt obliged to remain calm as the 'host' and for Sophie, who was my fiancée at the time and had accompanied me on this trip. She did not react well to the news and I did not want to add to her sense of panic. She was unfamiliar with the habit of multinational reorganizations and basically thought we were all being sacked!

The reality was that deep down I was worried and anxious and I had woken up earlier than usual because I felt uncertain about my situation: there were no guarantees and I would have to reapply for a job like everyone else. What I have come to realize is that my tendency to suppress my feelings meant that I often served as a container of others' worries and concerns. This could very well have created unconscious stressors that affected my sleep through the release of stress hormones such as adrenaline, thus stimulating the waking centre of my brain and stopping me from sleeping.

Delving into the analysis of my emotions at the time, I can now see that my tendency to maintain a calm façade was my typical coping response. Two possible explanations for my 'reflex' calmness are genetic predisposition and the lack of parrhesia or 'frankness of speech'. Both my mother and my father tended to 'contain' a lot of emotions, projecting something of a stoic attitude even when they were worried about personal or professional issues through-out our childhood. In replicating this behaviour in my adulthood, I recognized that I viewed this stoic attitude in a favourable light unconsciously. I would also attribute my predisposition to growing up in a very polite atmosphere and not speaking up. It encouraged me to conform rather than to assert my perspectives. This testified to one of the key aspects of Kets de Vries' clinical paradigm:[1] people are influenced by significant caregivers during their formative years. Working in a corporate environment that encouraged conformity, particularly among younger employees, only augmented my tendency to suppress my true feelings.

The reality was that deep down I was worried and anxious and I had woken up earlier than usual because I felt uncertain about my situation.

CHAPTER 6:
FORMATION OF
SLEEP HABITS
(CHILDHOOD TO UNIVERSITY YEARS)

In this chapter I will present a chronological narrative of my sleep experiences from the early days until I started to experience real sleep issues. This will demonstrate how these challenges can sneak up on you, with additional details on how more sleep – in this case, in the form of naps – can improve performance and wellbeing for the individual.

Based on my initial recollections of the years dating from my earliest memories (when I was about three years old) to my entry into the working world at 22, sleep was a routine I thought little of. It was just something I experienced. What is of note about this period is that I probably developed entrenched sleep habits such as daytime napping and a predisposition towards waking up early as a result of this formative period.

Naps had been an integral part of my lifestyle since childhood. By the time I was four, I had already developed a habit of napping at the kindergarten. In fact, it was encouraged. Every day at around 10.30am we had something called 'heads down' where all the kids were asked to sit at a table and put their heads on their folded arms on the desk in front of them, no doubt so the teachers could have a tea break. I invariably slept for a few minutes then. Similarly, my parents, who took regular naps after lunch, also encouraged my siblings and me to either follow suit or keep quiet so as not to wake them. I had thus been conditioned from a young age to view daytime naps as a 'normal' part of life.

The habit of waking up early – setting the alarm to ring 30–60 minutes earlier than my previous time to wake up for school in order to catch up on school work or prepare for a test – started when I was almost ten years old. This practice stemmed from a tip my dad had passed on to me regarding how to prepare for a make-up test at school. He advised me to get up about an hour before the usual time to study – when it is quiet and my mind would be clear. This strategy worked on that first occasion – with the early morning swotting I triumphed with an exhilarating result and came second in the class! Feeling that I was onto a winner, I carried this habit into my adolescence and university years, sleeping less than the usual eight hours when I had to meet an assignment deadline. However, at the time, given my youth and the infrequency of these episodes, these late nights did not seem to affect me unduly.

Hence, at this phase of my life I was able to recover swiftly, typically via afternoon naps – at least an hour, often up to two hours – to feel adequately rested in order to participate in my daily life. I could nap anywhere, especially on the coach heading home after college, and I was proud of it! Thus, this period turned out to be pivotal in planting the seeds of my habitual tendency to exchange sleep for work.

"

Studies have demonstrated ... strategic naps can be used effectively to promote performance and alertness in operational settings.

"

NASA report

THE BENEFITS OF TAKING A NAP

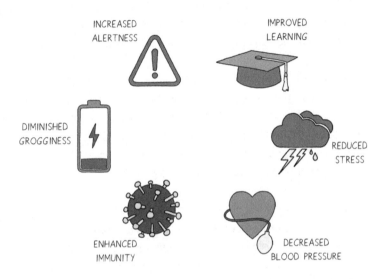

INCREASED
ALERTNESS

IMPROVED
LEARNING

DIMINISHED
GROGGINESS

REDUCED
STRESS

ENHANCED
IMMUNITY

DECREASED
BLOOD PRESSURE

Naps have always helped me mitigate a poor night's sleep, almost like a second chance allowing me to upgrade the night! Various studies have shown the benefits of napping. According to research from the Sorbonne University in Paris, short naps can reduce stress and enhance the immune system. According to one of the authors, Bruce Feraut, "Our data suggests a 30-minute nap can reverse the hormonal impact of a night of poor sleep."[1]

In addition, a study at Allegheny College, Pennsylvania showed that napping for 45 minutes a day helped lower blood pressure in those completing a stressful activity compared to those who hadn't.[2] This aligns with data from Greece showing that a sample of people taking regular noontime naps had a 5% decrease in blood pressure. This may seem small, but it's sufficient to reduce the incidence of heart attacks.[3]

NASA has long been interested in sleep in general, and naps in particular, for obvious reasons. According to one of their reports, "Studies have demonstrated ... strategic naps can be used effectively to promote performance and alertness in operational settings."[4]

One fascinating study from Saarland University in Germany showed the potential of naps to increase learning power. Students learned words both singularly and in pairs. After this, half the group watched a DVD, the other half napped. Afterwards they were tested on what they'd retained and those who'd napped showed "a five-fold improvement in information retrieval from memory."[5]

Some of the above cognitive benefits can be linked to a study by Georgetown University Medical Centre. Here, they reported that while napping, the right side of the brain, often linked to creativity, was highly active, with the left side much quieter.[6] And great news for those of us over 50 years of age, where research into older adults in Japan showed that, when combined with moderate exercise, a 30-minute nap can improve the quality of sleep at night and reduce grogginess in the day.[7]

And why nap rather than dose yourself with sugar and/or caffeine? In what is to me a particularly insightful study, Sara Mednick, Professor of Psychology at the University of California, Riverside, compared the relative beneficial effects on memory and problem-solving of 200mg of caffeine (roughly what we get from a cup of coffee). They had equal benefit to perceptual learning; however, naps outscored caffeine in word recall and motor learning (which apparently was actually weakened by caffeine).[8]

CHAPTER 7:
STILL CRUISING
THROUGH SLEEP ...
ALMOST
(EARLY TO MIDDLE ADULTHOOD)

Despite the fact that I did not experience any debilitating sleep difficulties throughout my early to middle adulthood, my failure to set
proper boundaries with regards to work had its origins during this
period. My work requirements and accompanying work schedules
would come to play an increasingly intrusive role in shaping my
lifestyle and eat into my sleeping hours.

Sleeping at about 11pm and waking up at 7am, what deviated from
the norm were my daytime naps. When I was 23–25, I drove at least
200 kilometres per day, four or five days a week, in my work as a
salesman in the UK. Typically experiencing drowsiness after lunch
during my work week, I would take a 20–30-minute nap. When I
awoke, I often felt a surge of energy that would power me through
to night time. I would feel so alert at night that I would work on my
computer in my home office, sometimes until midnight, to catch up
on the day's administrative work. And while there are some widespread observations about the potential negative effect of napping
making it harder for people to initiate sleep at night, I am still all
for naps – it's just that I've learned that to get the best out of them
you need to be quite strategic as to how and when you take them.

With the launch of my global career in a multinational corporation, I flew with increasing frequency across multiple time zones. Over a six-year period, I travelled almost monthly from London to Africa, and then to South and Central Asia where the time zones were 2–6 hours ahead of the time at home. However, all it would take was an extra two-hour nap for me to fully recover from the effects of jet lag. Therefore, during this phase of my life, I fell into the category of sleepers that fall asleep easily. My ability to rebound from the effects of jet lag during my young adult phase can be explained by the relative higher level of sleep efficiency of young adults compared to their older selves.

When in my early 30s, I was posted to Ho Chi Minh City in Vietnam, where I lived for almost four years. Work began to intrude even further into my life: during the first 18 months, I worked for 12 hours, six days a week. Even after work, I would be socializing with fellow expatriate colleagues and their families, talking shop late into the evening. Although my sleep was still not affected, I was plagued by a mysterious health problem over those 18 months. Suffering from recurring symptoms of dizziness, vertigo, loss of balance, nausea and vomiting, I was invalided back to the UK in April 1997 where I was diagnosed with benign paroxysmal positional vertigo (BPPV) – an inner ear problem leading to a spinning sensation caused by changes in the position of the head. The UK specialist informed me that my episodes of BPPV would decline significantly if I worked less and relaxed more. Working less and socializing with a more varied group of people meant that I talked less about work, and only two more BPPV episodes ensued thereafter. While my affliction seemed unrelated to my sleep patterns, it was significant in illuminating the first sign of the adverse impact of excessive work on my health.

Nonetheless, after recovering from BPPV I led an active social life that reduced my sleep from seven to six hours a night over the next two years. I would make up for this loss of sleep by napping in the car for 30–45 minutes during the working day whenever the opportunity presented itself, as I was often being driven to client meetings in different parts of Vietnam. However, I would still feel tired and low in energy after lunch, relying on coffee and walks around the office compound to stay awake. I would also try to catch up on my sleep with 1–2-hour naps at weekends. My fatigue and low energy after lunch thus indicated that my lifestyle of staying out until close to midnight and getting up at 6am was catching up with me.

When I look back on my work lifestyle, the BPPV and the emerging signs of sleep issues during my 30s, I wonder why I did not adjust my lifestyle to take my health issues more seriously. At the unconscious level, I could have been suppressing my stress from work. In my well-paid position as an expatriate leader, I often concealed how worried I was about the business from my Vietnamese national team. One possible psychodynamic concept that could account for my attitude is psychological containment – the capacity to internally manage troubling thoughts and feelings that arise from stress. My 'reflex' to contain my stress was something I had probably picked up from my parents during my childhood. They rarely showed strong negative emotions in front of us, sending us to our rooms if they had a difficult issue to discuss. At school, we were similarly encouraged to keep control and remain calm. I carried this attitude into my work as an adult.

The psychodynamic concept of a 'hidden competing commitment' could also be relevant. I had an improvement goal: to achieve a better balance in my life so that I would not get sick again. However, while I cut back on work, I replaced it with a very intense social life. I was out almost every night, often consuming more alcohol than was good for me. Applying the hidden competing commitments analysis revealed my biggest discomfort, or outright fear, driving me to do the opposite of what I was saying was the behaviour I wanted. In truth, like most people I had a strong need for love and belonging. I was lonely in Vietnam and in denial about it. I threw everything into my job and social life, so that I would not have the time or the energy to reflect on the rest of my life. Sound familiar?

I've learned that to get the best out of them, you need to be quite strategic as to how and when you take [naps].

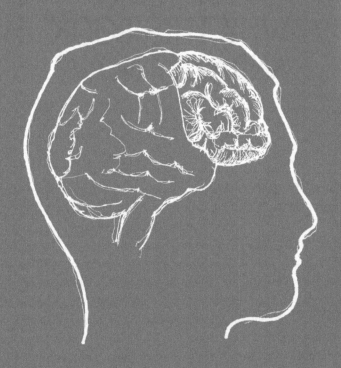

PART TWO

WHAT IS SLEEP?

CHAPTER 8:
WHY THIS BOOK
AND WHY NOW?

Among the growing literature on sleep in recent years there have been multiple books and articles exploring the function of sleep, the challenges we experience in sleeping, plus some tips to address the nightmare of sleep deprivation. These books and articles are typically written by academics or medical doctors with an in-depth knowledge of the subject. What they often lack, however, is a personal experience of chronic sleep deprivation over a sustained period of time and the resulting impact it can have on an individual's personal and professional life. That's where *Positive Sleep* fits in; a book by a layman who had major sleep challenges and was able to overcome them through trial and error. I've already given a brief yet comprehensive, holistic and compelling exploration of the effects of the chronic sleep problems I suffered from. I will seek to help you understand why the issue of sleep is – literally – a matter of life and death and what you can do about it.

So if I am able to trigger a dialogue between individuals and organizations to take the steps required to address this debilitating phenomenon, then I will feel the two-fingered tapping away at the keyboard to write this book will have been worthwhile! After all, you will feel (and problem solve) so much better after a good night's sleep.

As for 'why now'? Well it appears that the sleep deprivation epidemic is simply getting worse and worse. At least 75 health issues have been connected with poor sleep, including evidence showing a link to Alzheimer's. In fact, even just a few consecutive days of sleep deprivation can make our responses comparable to being drunk.

Conservative estimates suggest that on average in the UK and the US, we are getting between one and two hours less sleep than we were in the 1950s. Now, could it be that since this time we've evolved to such an extent as humans that we no longer need 7–8 hours sleep in a 24-hour period? I doubt it. What is far more likely is that the pressures and opportunities to do things other than sleep have grown exponentially since then. From the widespread impact of television, through to the age of globalization and to the dawn of social media and smartphones, the 'I'll sleep when I'm dead' mentality has become explicitly or implicitly widespread. Many people simply have no clue of the harm they are doing to themselves.

It is as if, regardless of their significance, all of these activities are being categorized into what the late Stephen Covey used to call the "Urgent and Important" box.

CHAPTER 9:
WHY WE SLEEP
DIFFERENTLY –
HOW AGE IMPACTS THIS

While there is no definitive research to explain why we sleep, there is significant evidence to indicate that sleep is critical in enabling both our bodies, and especially our brains, to recharge. Sleep bolsters the functioning of the brain in the following ways. First, sleep can 'restore the energy' used by the brain for reflection. Second, it enables the brain to 'reorder and store' the important information acquired during the day. Third, sufficient sleep is also needed for the development of 'new brain cells' that are important in long-term memory.[1]

Based on the function of sleep for recharging the mind, it is evident that sleep deprivation can have a plethora of adverse consequences. I'll address the physiological, cognitive, emotional and social consequences of sleep deprivation later in the book, along with the good news – what everyone can do about it.

To understand why we sleep differently – and what age has to do with it – we need a basic understanding (and I do mean basic!) of what determines when we sleep and when we wake up. There are two forces at work here. The first is typically known as the circadian clock, sometimes described as the circadian rhythm or body clock. The second is a chemical in your brain called adenosine that creates pressure to sleep.

The first force – the circadian clock – is generated internally, as Kleitman and Richardson showed in their 1938 experiment and as described in detail by Matthew Walker in his book *Why We Sleep?*[2] In what was then groundbreaking sleep research, the researchers lived in a cave for weeks and showed that this clock is not light dependent, yet exists within us. Without exposure to the sun signalling day and night, they morphed into a routine of typically being awake for 15 hours and sleeping for approximately 9 hours over a 24-hour period. Since this research, further study has helped us to understand that this circadian rhythm in humans is normally slightly over 24 hours; however, daylight adjusts this in humans and other living species primarily through a part of our brain which also controls our body temperature.

Yet how can that be? We know people who describe themselves as either 'night owls' or 'morning larks' – I'm firmly in the latter camp, with the whole of this book being written in the morning as that's my best time. So, if you are finding this book dull so far, Lord knows what it would have been like if I'd written it in the evening!

It turns out that it's not our fault if we are bright-eyed and alert in the morning, or if we come to life more in the evening. This preference is strongly determined by our genetics – another thing we can blame our parents for! This is tough on night owls; in some societies they can be seen as lazy as they struggle to get up early. And if they are forced to work a traditional 9-5 day, they can end up being sleep deprived. Matthew Walker describes this succinctly, writing that "it's not their conscious fault, rather their genetic fate." What makes this even tougher is that this lack of sleep results in a greater chance of ill health, specifically higher incidences of depression, anxiety, diabetes, cancer, heart attacks and strokes.[3]

So, what internal signals indicate to our body that it's time to sleep? Well, a part of the brain (called the suprachiasmatic nucleus) signals this via the release of a hormone called melatonin. Released from the back of the brain – the pineal gland to be precise – it's the signal for the timing of sleep. Humans receive the first waves of this in the evening, whereas nocturnal creatures such as bats and foxes get this message in the morning. You can think of it as the green light rather than the generator of sleep, normally kicking in after dark and declining in production throughout the night until about 4am.

So that's the first force, the circadian clock and its messenger melatonin. The second force can be called sleep pressure. This is the result of the chemical I mentioned called adenosine building up in the brain every minute you are awake. As we will discuss later, caffeine has the opposite effect, masking adenosine and fighting to keep you awake.

These two forces – the circadian rhythm and the chemical adenosine – do not cooperate. They are distinct, separate systems, though they typically align their functions. They help us to have strong urges to sleep and wake up on a reasonably regular rhythm when uninterrupted by caffeine, jet lag and other shocks to the sleep system which I'll come to later.

A common perception is that age also has an impact on why we sleep differently, and this is correct. From what we've learned from mid-20th century sleep research, this seems driven by our need for different types of sleep as distinguished below.

Sleep can be determined through three types of activity – brainwaves, eye movements and muscles. In 1952, through using this data, Nathaniel Kleitman – our man from the cave experiment in the late 1930s – and Eugene Aserinsky noticed distinct variations in eye movements, and that these variations seemed to occur in patterns throughout the night.[4] These distinct sleep phases were named Non-Rapid Eye Movement (NREM) sleep and Rapid Eye Movement (REM) sleep. We now know that we sleep in approximately 90-minute cycles, commencing and ending with REM sleep and with different depths of NREM sleep in between. We'll come back to these stages in more detail later. However, for now it's important to note that NREM sleep is a relaxation mode for the brain, especially the cortex, a sort of nocturnal cerebral meditation, a time of 'reflection and storing.' By contrast, REM sleep prompts 'integration,' an upgrading of the way we view how the world works, and augmenting our capacity for insight and problem-solving.

NREM VS REM SLEEP

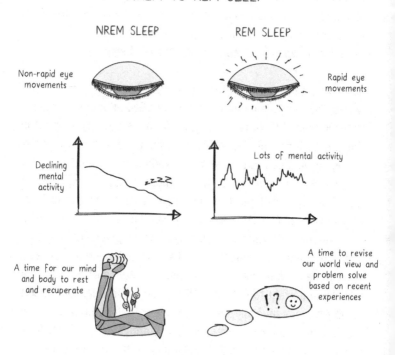

NREM SLEEP

Non-rapid eye movements

Declining mental activity

zzzz

A time for our mind and body to rest and recuperate

REM SLEEP

Rapid eye movements

Lots of mental activity

A time to revise our world view and problem solve based on recent experiences

!?☺

This brief glimpse into what happens when we sleep provides information that can help us understand how we sleep differently throughout our lives, as this is driven in part by the type of sleep we need.

There is evidence to suggest that most unborn babies sleep most of the time – partly REM sleep, partly NREM sleep and the rest a state somewhere in between these two. A bias towards REM sleep is then observed in the final trimester, plus a small window of a couple of hours when the baby is awake.

So, what internal
signals indicate
to our body
that it's time
to sleep?

In the early weeks after birth, infants sleep in small doses totaling as much as 16 hours in a 24-hour period.[5] At six months a baby typically sleeps 14 hours a day, with an approximately 50:50 split of NREM:REM. The richness of these early months in REM sleep supports the brain development of the neural pathways and connections. At the age of one an infant typically sleeps mostly at night, and by the age of four they typically need just one nap per day.

At five years old, kids typically sleep for approximately 11 hours per day, and the split shifts to 70:30 NREM:REM as the deep sleep reflection and storing qualities become increasingly called for. This becomes even more important in teenagers, and there appears to be a link to this deep sleep emphasis and the development of cognitive skills, reasoning and critical thinking as the brain further matures. However, as most parents of adolescents will tell you, there is a shift in the body clock of the average teenager such that they wish to stay up later and wake up later. This appears to be the result of a genuine – if temporary – shift in their circadian rhythm, which often leads to parental conflict!

As we mature through our twenties and throughout the rest of our lives, there is a common view that we need less sleep to function. However, research suggests this is not the case; it's merely that both the quality and quantity of our sleep worsens throughout these years. There are many reasons for this including the fact that ageing results in a weaker bladder function and, eventually, after a certain age we will always have an interrupted night because we need to use the bathroom. There is also a shift in circadian rhythms so we need to sleep earlier (not ideal if you have teenagers in the house!).

It's worth devoting a paragraph to the menopause, however, as this is something that I am asked about constantly. And from what I've read, Lockley and Foster sum this up best: "Menopause has major effects on sleep, inducing symptoms that affect sleep including night sweats and mood disorders, in addition to long sleep latencies and reduced slow-wave sleep. Post-menopausal women have nearly double the rate of insomnia complaints as pre-menopausal women, although when sleep is measured objectively, these differences are reversed, suggesting that hormonal status may also affect sleep-state misconception. Obstructive Sleep Apnea risk is three times higher after the menopause, most likely due to hormone-related redistribution of fat, and this appears to be reduced in women taking hormone replacement therapy (HRT)."[6]

Matthew Walker, in his book *Why We Sleep*, brings together decades of his own academic research and reading into a remarkable book that's almost encyclopedic in scope, yet readable in style and length. I recommend this to you if the above has sparked your interest sufficiently to want to dig further.

CHAPTER 10:
HOW DO WE
DEFINE SLEEP

Every night we undergo a remarkable change. We leave waking consciousness and for hours we sleep, and sometimes dream too. We rarely think about or appreciate that we are sleeping while we are asleep and when we wake up we typically remember little about our sleep.

Hence, although everyone sleeps, defining sleep is quite another matter. From observing changes in behaviour and our reactions when asleep, scientists such as those at the Harvard Medical School (http://healthysleep.med.harvard.edu/) have provided the following definitions for sleep:[1]

- A phase of the day when activity drops right down compared to the balance of the 24 hours.
- Associated with a habitual posture; in the case of humans this is typically lying down with closed eyes.
- When we are asleep we are less reactive to external stimuli.
- Unlike hibernation and being in a coma, we can reverse the state of sleep relatively easily.

Additionally, from observing behavioural changes that accompany sleep and the physiological changes linked to this, scientists now define sleep in humans primarily based on brainwave activity patterns, plus some other physiological changes.

CHAPTER 11: SLEEP AND PHYSIOLOGY

THE ARCHITECTURE OF SLEEP

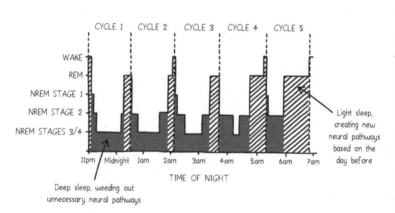

Deep sleep, weeding out unnecessary neural pathways

Light sleep, creating new neural pathways based on the day before

During the day we need certain aspects of our body to be relatively constant, or at least tightly controlled, so that we can optimize performance of the task at hand. This includes our glucose, CO_2 and oxygen levels, plus temperature and blood pressure that are routinely checked when we visit a doctor.

However, during a night's sleep, we don't have the same physiological needs. Hence our body temperature and blood pressure normally drop. In NREM sleep our brain activity, heartbeat and breathing are typically quite regular, however this becomes much more variable during REM sleep, which is much closer to the pattern observed when we are awake.

Different physiological activities behave differently while we sleep. For example, urine production falls along with the slowing of kidney activity. Conversely, it has been estimated that as much as 75% of human growth hormone is released during sleep.[1] Furthermore, the amount of cell repair that goes on suggests it may well be an important function of sleep.

OUR BRAIN

Until relatively recently, the consensus was that the brain was inactive during sleep. However, since the since the mid-20th century we have known that the opposite is true. As the Havard Medical School describes it, "There is a progressive decrease or 'firing' rate of most neurons throughout the brain as sleep progresses from wakefulness to non-REM sleep. Also, the patterns of neuron firing change from a seemingly random and variable activity pattern during wakefulness, to a much more coordinated and synchronous pattern during non-REM sleep."[2]

We have also learnt the most common characteristics and patterns of sleep, as well as how significant medicine, disease, our own lifestyle and other factors can shape our sleep quality and quantity. And we are aware that during REM sleep "there is an increase in firing rate of most neurons throughout the brain, as compared to non-REM sleep."[3] In fact, the brain in REM sleep may at times be even more active than when we are awake! This is widely assumed to be linked to the intense, colourful dreams that can take place during REM sleep.

One point of interest which the Harvard Medical School alerts us to is that "when humans sleep, the entire brain is involved. Dolphins and whales, on the other hand, need to maintain consciousness while they sleep so they can occasionally surface to breathe. In these marine mammals, sleep occurs in only one hemisphere of their brain at a time – allowing for some degree of consciousness and vigilance to be maintained at all times."[4]

OUR BODY

Through a process known as thermoregulation, the temperature of our body is controlled by mechanisms such as shivering and sweating to minimize variation throughout the day. Then, prior to sleeping our body starts to lose heat, which may actually help us to sleep. During sleep, our body temperature drops circa 1°C, falling furthest during REM sleep. Hence the use of a blanket!

Thus we use less energy to maintain our body temperature, prompting some scientists to put forward the view that conserving energy may be one of the primary functions of sleep.

"
When humans sleep, the entire brain is involved.

"

Harvard Medical School

OUR BREATHING

Our breathing patterns vary between being awake and being asleep. While awake there is no set pattern to our breathing, it is a function of what we are doing – speaking, running etc. – and how we are feeling. Much like our brain pattern, our breathing in NREM sleep slows down and becomes relatively predictable. And once in REM sleep, there's an increase in breathing rate, almost as if we are awake.

OUR HEART

Giving our heart the chance to rest may well be a function of sleep. During NREM sleep both our heart rate and blood pressure drop. The opposite is observed during REM sleep. The root causes of these variations during REM sleep are seemingly unknown, though the Harvard Medical School suggests this "may be a by-product of REM-related changes in nervous system activity or related dream content."[5]

OUR DREAMS

Dreaming occurs in both REM and NREM sleep. And if you think we've still got plenty to learn about what sleep is, try studying the available literature on dreams! We typically understand dreaming to be a time when our thoughts follow bizarre and seemingly illogical sequences. Sometimes they feel random, at other times they seem linked to our experiences during daytime. REM-sleep is most widely linked to dreaming, when our most visually intense dreams happen. Moreover, research suggests that nightmares occur during NREM sleep.

Despite a myriad of literature espousing different hypotheses to explain dreams, there appears to be no consensus thus far. One unproven theory is that dreams represent a re-run of the day's events to enable these to form into memories. Others see dreams existing purely as the result of random activity in the brain.

However, in his book *Why We Sleep*, Matthew Walker pulls together various strands of research to propose the idea that REM sleep plus dreaming combine to serve two purposes: "The first function involves nursing our emotional and mental health ... The second is problem solving and creativity."[6]

Having worked through – based on the available research – what sleep is, we can now look at the cost of poor sleep in different ways.

CHAPTER 12:
SLEEP DEPRIVATION
AND PHYSIOLOGY

A key physiological consequence of sleep deprivation is the development of sleep disorders. Estimates vary as to how many physical ailments can be attributed to poor sleep. However, somewhere in the region of 75 distinct illnesses seems a fair assumption based on the data. I have personal experience of two of the most common – insomnia and sleep-related breathing disorders. In addition, my struggle with sleep deprivation was also accompanied by a related problem – obesity.

INSOMNIA

The most common sleep complaint is insomnia – a broad symptom describing the inability to sleep. I suffered primarily from sleep-maintenance insomnia – being able to fall asleep easily but not stay asleep, and then waking up too early. This is distinct from sleep onset insomnia, when nodding off itself is tough. For some it's transient and associated with a particular life event, whereas for others it feels like a permanent and apparently insoluble battle.

Up to 40% of adults may suffer from insomnia at some time in their lives, with 15% experiencing chronic insomnia. The three main causes are: first, an inherent disposition; second, some major trigger or shock to the system such as a major life event (for example, a birth or death, a marriage or divorce); and finally, a series of behaviours that amplify insomnia: e.g. using smartphones, tablets and computers just before bedtime, eating or exercising late, too much caffeine consumption or napping at the wrong time.

Untreated insomnia is linked to numerous health problems, the only real debate sometimes being whether the insomnia causes the health issue or the other way around! However, insomnia has been shown to have a strong link to an increased risk of heart disease, stroke and depression, plus various psychiatric disorders.

SLEEP-RELATED BREATHING DISORDERS

Another classification of sleep disorders is sleep-related breathing disorders, which manifested in me in the form of sleep apnoea and snoring. Obstructive sleep apnoea (OSA) is characterized by the repeated partial or complete closing of the airway during sleep, thus cutting off the air supply. As it causes suffocation and abrupt awakening, sleep apnoea prevents individuals from falling into deep sleep. This is why sufferers are typically very tired during the day.

The sound emitted during snoring is caused by a partial blockage at any point from the tip of the nose to the vocal chords. Snoring leads to the loss of sleep when the snorer wakes others who, in turn, rouse the snorer. I first became very conscious of this on a skiing holiday in my early twenties. So bad was my snoring, plus the dramatic-sounding pauses in my breathing which sounded life threatening, that my three fellow skiers would take it in turns to share a twin room with me. The sleep tests I had suggested that my apnoea was mild. For those who have severe sleep apnoea, they may well stop breathing 30 times per hour, and in the most severe cases it can be 100 times per hour.

This sleep disruption can stop sufferers from sleeping deeply enough, hence they become very tired and simply cannot concentrate. This is a common cause of driving accidents as a result of drowsy driving. Waking up every few minutes – even only for a matter of seconds – makes the heart rate more variable, raises blood pressure and increases the risk of strokes and heart attacks, plus there is an increased risk of diabetes.

OBESITY

Another physiological factor that is associated with sleep disorders is obesity. Researchers suggest that chronic sleep deprivation may produce weight gain, either by increasing food intake or decreasing the energy burnt. It's also been found that sleep deprivation can increase the levels of hormones that stimulate appetite and decrease the levels of hormones that induce satiety, so that you are simply hungrier the less you sleep.[1] There is also a significantly increased chance of developing Type 2 diabetes.[2]

Certainly, I do not crave food to the same extent now that I sleep better. And a detox from alcohol, all dairy products and carbohydrates had a positive effect on my sleep by helping me to lose weight and clean up my gut. However, the reverse can be true too – should I go through even a few days where, for whatever reason, my sleep is disturbed and I am not getting the 7.5–8 hours I regard as ideal, then I want to eat more, and my first thoughts are not for a plate of broccoli!

For the sake of completeness, in addition to insomnia and sleep-related breathing disorders, which are the most common, here are the others based on the International Classification of Sleep Disorders (ICSD-2):

Hypersomnia of central origin is excessive daytime sleepiness. Hypersomnia is not due to sleep apnoea – as in my case – but is a central disorder in the brain. Narcolepsy is the best known of the three types of this disorder, also known as sleep attacks, when you simply must sleep even if you've been quite active seconds before. This must be terrifying for the less than 0.2% of the population that suffer from it. The other types of this disorder are idiopathic hypersomnia (daytime sleepiness for no apparent reason) and recurrent hypersomnia (recurring bouts of daytime sleepiness and other cognitive dysfunction).[3]

Circadian rhythm sleep disorders occur when wanting to sleep at times that are not aligned with the usual circadian cycle. Groups most commonly affected include adolescents, the elderly, the blind and some dementia patients. Treatments normally involve resetting the timing of sleep to its proper place in the circadian cycle through the use of light and melatonin at precise times and in strict doses.

Lockyer and Foster describe **parasomnias** as "undesirable events that occur 'alongside sleep'."[4] Examples include nightmares, sleepwalking and bed-wetting. Parasomnias, at their most extreme, can sometimes prove dangerous to both sufferers and their sleeping partners.

Up to 40% of adults may suffer from insomnia at some time in their lives, with 15% experiencing chronic insomnia.

Sleep-related movement disorders include restless legs syndrome (RLS). This can occur when awake as well as when asleep, and when you've been at rest for some time. According to Lockyer and Foster it's more common in women than men.

In addition, there are **isolated symptoms and normal variants and other sleep disorders** which represent the miscellaneous bucket![5]

CHAPTER 13: SLEEP AND COGNITION

The impact of sleep deprivation on cognitive performance may be slightly more hidden than the physiological impacts. However, to many this is arguably even more important.

To be able to maintain one's focus on results, individuals have to be able to keep their eye on the ball and avoid distractions, while at the same time ensuring that they (and their businesses) are heading in the right direction. Several well-regarded studies reveal how cognitive performance declines with excessive wakefulness. One study in particular showed that staying awake for 17–19 hours and more was equivalent to being in a 'drunken' state. The performance of different individuals across a range of activities was shown to be similar to someone with a blood-alcohol level of 0.05%, the legal driving limit in some countries.[1] In another study, where the effects of chronic sleep restriction were studied, it was found that cognitive performance after 14 consecutive days of six hours of sleep or less appeared to have the same effect as two nights without any sleep. However, even more worrying is that the people undergoing such sleep studies often cannot perceive the declines in their own cognitive performance, and this goes some way to explain why people are unaware that their sleep deprivation is undermining their ability to work.

To continue with the effects that are especially significant in the business world, problem-solving is another that encompasses diverse cognitive functions – insight, pattern recognition and one's ability to be innovative and creative. It can be severely affected by cutting corners on sleep, the sort of behaviour that is all too common in those in leadership positions who need these skills and behaviours the most. The converse is also true. Sufficient sleep not only enables people to identify solutions, but also promotes their ability to integrate information and come up with creative ideas.

One further critical leadership behaviour is the ability to evaluate the viability of different perspectives. Sleep exerts a positive impact on the ability to assimilate new information, which is important for evaluating new ideas. This cognitive ability is vital for leaders to accurately evaluate the relative significance of different inputs and reduce cognitive bias. Complex cognitive-emotional decision-making, where emotional responses and financial risk and rewards need to be integrated, would also be enhanced by sufficient sleep. From personal experience, I know how, when you're tired, you're often tempted to disregard the opinions of others and simply focus on 'getting the job done.' Such shortsightedness may well come back and harm you in the longer term.

CHAPTER 14: SOCIAL AND EMOTIONAL WELLBEING

The lack of sleep can also undermine your ability to maintain emotional stability. The impact of sleep deprivation on emotional dimensions is also of great importance to anyone in an organization, especially the leaders, and also those in the caring professions. One of the keys in both roles is the ability to support others. The first critical step to support others is to understand them. One common way to do this is to accurately interpret the emotions conveyed in their tone of voice or facial expressions. Research shows that even one single night of sleep deprivation affects our ability to recognize human facial emotional intensities.

The specific negative emotional effects of sleep deprivation can also interfere with our social interactions. When you are short of sleep, there is a significantly higher chance that your brain will misinterpret what's happening and overreact, particularly to stressful or challenging situations.

Sleep deprivation, particularly due to sleep conditions that could disrupt the sleep of others, can also place social relationships under pressure. For instance, sleep apnoea causes the sufferer to wake up with a noisy gasp that is typically startling, enough to cause a bed partner to wake up. Snoring can also disturb the sleep of others. In the long term, the disruptive effects of such sleep conditions can lead to couples sleeping apart. A National Sleep Foundation survey, 2010 *Sleep in America*, found that 23% of couples slept apart due to snoring and other sleep-related issues. A similar number also reported that their intimate relationships had been affected because they were too sleepy to engage in sexual activity.

CHAPTER 15:
EVOLUTION OF
SLEEP THROUGH
LIFE PHASES

In studying the development of sleep difficulties over a lifespan, it can be seen that an individual's sleep habits and patterns, as well as the body's need for sleep and ability to recover from lack of sleep, will evolve through various life phases. Just focusing on an individual's struggle with sleep issues within a short time frame, therefore, will not offer a comprehensive portrait of their changing struggle with sleep throughout an entire lifetime.

To begin with, the family of origin plays a critical role in shaping sleep habits. Sleep habits, established in early childhood, can form the foundation of sleep practices for the rest of a person's life. The first sleep habit is not related so much to sleep but to the formation of work habits that affect one's sleep. Based on their evaluation of diverse research studies, Whitebread and Bingham[1] found that parenting styles and practices are important in shaping children's attitudes towards learning and work habits. For instance, the positive association of waking up early to do work during an individual's childhood can lead to the adult habit of sleeping less to get up early to do work. As I mentioned, this is something I suffered from for decades and still have to guard against now. The adverse impact of sleep deprivation can become obscured by the adult's perception that this reduction of sleep is justified because it has been 'sacrificed' for work.

Literature has highlighted the potential benefits of a second habit, napping, with specific information on the optimal duration and timing. I remember reading about how NASA had researched sleep extensively to help their astronauts optimize their time in space, 26 minutes being the ideal time quoted. Not 25 or 27 minutes – 26 minutes! However, it has a downside: napping could be a primary or partial contributor to individuals experiencing fatigue when waking up in the morning or having difficulties falling or staying asleep.

This has played out in my own case where I acquired lifelong habits through my upbringing of waking up early to work and napping.

The issue with these sleep habits is that they often become an entrenched part of your lifestyle before the occurrence of sleep difficulties, typically in later adulthood. As mentioned earlier, our sleep patterns evolve significantly as we grow older in terms of how we fall and remain asleep. Furthermore, our ability to have seven to eight hours of uninterrupted sleep declines. The overall trend is that the older we get, the lower our sleep efficiency; essentially, we have a tendency to sleep less and wake up earlier. While waking up during the night may occur with young adults, there seems to be a protective mechanism at play, which prevents them from waking up fully. The effectiveness of this mechanism begins to decrease as we grow older: research has shown that between the ages of 20 and 60, our slow-wave sleep (SWS), or deep sleep, falls at a rate of about 2% per decade.

The overall trend is that the older we get, the lower our sleep efficiency.

This goes some way to explaining why older adults are more likely to experience difficulties with sleep, as these issues begin to surface with age. However, the underlying issues that have contributed to their sleep problems would have been years in the making or related to their life phase.

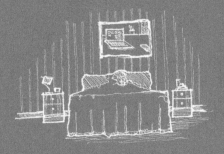

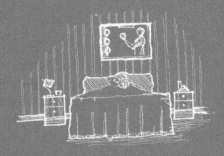

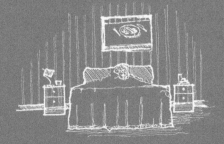

IMPACT OF SLEEP

CHAPTER 16:
SOCIETAL ATTITUDES
TOWARDS SLEEP

Struggles with sleep difficulties have been further exacerbated by society's failure to recognize the seriousness of sleep issues and their adverse effects on individuals, their families, their organizations and society as a whole. Sleep expert David K Randall put it succinctly in his book *Dreamland*: "Sleep remains ingrained in our cultural ethos as something that can be put off, dosed or ignored." Unlike our willingness to invest in healthy foods, exercise regimens and relaxing vacations in the pursuit of a healthy lifestyle, sleep is often pushed to the periphery. Apparently, putting one's head on the pillow is not regarded as taking an active step to improving your life.

This indifference towards the impact of sleep deprivation on work performance is also widespread within organizations. It remains a hidden issue among leaders as very few people are willing to admit that sleep deprivation is a problem among working professionals. As Theo Compernolle argued in his brilliant book *Brain Chains*, more than half of the professionals and managers attending his workshops or coaching sessions have become "used to the sleepiness of unhealthy low levels of sleep." They have deluded themselves into thinking that they belong to the approximately "15% of people who are genetically short sleepers, and who live healthy lives with seven hours of sleep or less."[1]

By not giving sleep issues a strong priority, the medical establishment is also a likely contributor to such societal attitudes. The subject is taught in a rather cursory fashion at medical schools, and hence the general level of teaching and understanding of sleep by doctors appears to be poor. There are complaints about doctors' abilities to address the sleep issues of their patients. In my own experience, I have also found that there are only a limited number of medically qualified sleep experts in the UK. In fact, as already mentioned, on one trip to my general practitioner I described my challenges with sleep. "You're lucky," he said, and proceeded on a monologue on his own inability to get to sleep at night.

After barely a moment's thought, when I'd left his surgery I placed the prescription he had given me for the drug temazepam in the bin outside.

The lack of 'seriousness' towards this medical problem is also reflected in the fact that not only is the UK National Health Service (NHS) not geared up to treat sleep issues, UK private health insurance does not provide insurance coverage for sleep conditions. This is something I discovered through my own experience. Thus, it would seem that the medical establishment needs to take the lead in overturning the current societal indifference towards sleep issues. This is very different in both the US and Australia, where you can get treatment for sleep issues through private health insurance.

"

Sleep remains ingrained in our cultural ethos as something that can be put off, dosed or ignored.

"

David K Randall,
author of *Dreamland*

CHAPTER 17: IMPACT OF LIFESTYLE ON SLEEP

While the quality of sleep can have an impact on our ability to work and relate to others, this is not a one-way relationship. Our responses to daily experiences can also affect the quality of our sleep. A hectic professional and personal lifestyle that incorporates multiple demands is one of the chief contributors to the poor quality of sleep.

In the 21st century, our use of technology is interwoven with the rest of our life and must rank up there with our attitude to work as a major impact on sleep. It can feel like we have the opportunity to connect with everybody and anybody merely through one click. As Arianna Huffington puts it elegantly " ... the never-ending possibility of connecting ... is, not surprisingly, addictive. Humans are social creatures – we are hard-wired to connect. Even when we're not actually connecting digitally, we're in a constant state of heightened anticipation. And always being in this state doesn't exactly put us in the right frame of mind to wind down when it's time to sleep. Though we don't give much thought to how we put ourselves to bed, we have little resting places and refueling shrines all over our houses, like little doll beds, where our technology can recharge, even if we can't."[1]

Being 'on call' at all times still seems a necessary condition for success. As Alan Derickson writes, "Sleep deprivation now resides within a repertoire of practices deemed essential to survival in a globally competitive world. More so than in the time of Thomas Edison, depriving oneself of necessary rest or denying it to those under one's control is considered necessary to success in a 24/7/365 society."[2]

Data from the US backs this up, where 30% of employees say they sleep less than six hours per night, and 70% per cent claim not to sleep enough.[3] Seeing these figures makes me wonder why we don't see even more cases of burnout than we do.

And there is also evidence to support the hypothesis that lower socio-economic groups suffer more, frequently working several jobs while often juggling childcare needs. A 2013 study from the University of Chicago found that "lower socio-economic position was associated with poorer subjective sleep quality, increased sleepiness and/or increased sleep complaints."[4] In addition, there appears to be a link between where you live (and the resulting stress) and how well you sleep. "I have never seen a study that hasn't shown a direct association between neighbourhood quality and sleep quality," said Lauren Hale, a Stony Brook University professor of preventative medicine.[5]

My personal view is that – in higher socio-economic groups and wealthier neighbourhoods – the tide may be finally turning here. As we will see later, elite sportsmen and women are starting to acknowledge sleep as a performance enhancer. This may yet prove to be a precursor to a wider lifestyle shift.

Elite sportsmen and women are starting to acknowledge sleep as a performance enhancer. This may yet prove to be a precursor to a wider lifestyle shift.

I truly hope so. In terms of my own experiences, I cannot say that lack of sleep cost me my marriage, for example. However, it certainly did not help; not just in my reduced ability to consider my wife's viewpoints, but also the consequences of my snoring and unusual nocturnal habits – sleeping by 9pm and leaping out of bed at 3am to work! Imagine being married to that!

CHAPTER 18:
IMPACT OF WORK
ON SLEEP

Working in a globalized economy with the requirement for frequent air travel to different regions can undermine sleep patterns significantly. Moreover, when the air travel takes place across time zones, working professionals will experience jet lag that disrupts their circadian clock. As already outlined, the circadian clock is a biological clock that drives us to be active in the day and to sleep at night within a circa 24-hour cycle.

Rapid travel from one region to another via jet planes does not provide sufficient time for the circadian clocks of travellers to adjust. "In other words, when we change time zones, we change sleep zones."[1] It can affect performance due to losses in concentration, attentiveness and reflective capacity. Researchers at Rush University Medical Centre in Chicago suggested jet lag could cause depression, gastric issues and affect one's judgement in the short-term, while affecting the menstrual cycle and our cognitive abilities in the longer term.[2]

Personally, I have lost count of the number of times I sat in meetings with senior leaders who wore their lack of sleep – after a flight from, say, Hong Kong to London – as a badge of honour. The truth was that not only were these so-called professionals effectively 'drunk at work' – such was their level of sleep deprivation – invariably, they also promptly started to nod off in meetings when not engaged in the conversation.

Fortunately, there are now multiple approaches that can be taken to alleviate this phenomena that has only truly been recognized since the early days of travel by jet. Starving yourself to get back onto a new clock is one approach, taking your own healthy snacks another. Although I rarely travel long distances on business these days, one technique that Arianna Huffington highlights particularly caught my eye, " ... an actual diet called the Argonne Anti-Jet-Lag Diet, named after the Argonne National Laboratory near Chicago, where it was formulated by the biologist Charles Ehret. With this method, four days before your trip you alternate two cycles of feasting and fasting, switching every two days, making sure to link up the last fasting day with the day you travel. The diet was tested in 2002 by U.S. National Guard troops going to and from South Korea. The anti-jet-lag group was 16.2 times less likely to experience jet lag on their way home from South Korea than the control group was."[3]

And for those that think that, despite these impressive looking statistics, the above diet looks like rather hard work and are not so keen on the many apps on the market, try the Re-Timer, "an eyeglasses-like piece of headwear that can be used ... by travelers ... Worn over the eyes, it exposes the wearer to a simulation of outdoor light, which, when used in the morning, can help reset our body clock so that we can fall asleep at the right bedtime."[4]

People fool themselves they can catch up at weekends for skimping on sleep during the week, while actually never recovering their sleep debt.

A colleague of mine, Marc Albas (a regular global traveller), swears by them as both effective and easy to use.

And it's not only travellers that are suffering the effects of a form of jet lag. Even more working professionals are affected by 'social jet lag' that is caused by the disparities between the sleep patterns of the weekend and the work week. Typically, working professionals sleep and wake up later during the weekend than the work week, often to compensate for the inadequate sleep they have experienced during the work week or due to social activities with friends. The shifting between these two sleep patterns disrupts the circadian clock that is essentially 'reset again on Monday.' This is extremely common in many societies – people fool themselves they can catch up at weekends for skimping on sleep during the week, while actually never recovering their sleep debt.

CHAPTER 19:
IMPACT OF DIET
AND EXERCISE
ON SLEEP

In addition to work, another big part of our lifestyle which can affect our sleep are the interrelated spheres of diet and exercise. One of the common beverages consumed by working professionals is coffee. Although the caffeine contained in coffee (and also in tea, some energy drinks, some chocolate, ice cream and some pills) can increase our reaction time and alertness, it exerts debilitating effects on sleep such as longer sleep latency, reduced sleep duration and suppressed slow-wave 'deep' sleep.

As mentioned earlier, adenosine is the chemical that accumulates in our brain as sleep pressure builds. Caffeine – a chemical that stimulates you – effectively blocks adenosine and hence the message does not get to the brain that it's time to sleep.

Caffeine also has a relatively long half-life: the amount of time needed to metabolize half the amount taken is five to seven hours. Therefore, a quarter of your intake at as early as 2pm could still be in your system at midnight to cause significant sleep disruption.

THE IMPACT OF DIET AND EXERCISE ON SLEEP

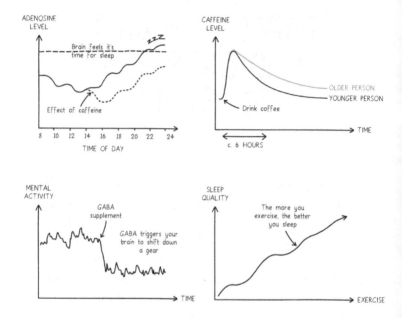

And it's well worth noting how we process caffeine to understand why people react differently to it. Caffeine is processed by an enzyme in the liver that becomes less effective as we age, and is also more efficient in some people than others. Hence our ability to do this is partially genetically related and the older we get, the harder we find it to process. Other medication we may be taking plus the quality and quantity of prior sleep can also be a factor.[1]

" Staying active won't cure sleep complaints ... but it will reduce the odds of them. "

Richard Dishman,
University of Georgia

Similarly, the consumption of alcohol is used by many to help them sleep. However, its effectiveness in facilitating sleep declines over time, not to mention the fact that its consumption disrupts sleep by causing an increased likelihood of 'nocturia' – urination at night.

The relationship between diet – and what goes on in your gut as a result – and sleep is quite complex. One example is the production in the gut of two key hormones – dopamine and GABA – which have both been found to impact sleep.

A group of Spanish researchers found that dopamine acts in the pineal gland, which is core to determining our circadian rhythm. They found these dopamine receptors only appear towards the end of the night, and are thought to be instrumental in stopping melatonin production when the day begins to start waking up the brain.[2]

GABA – the short name for gamma-Aminobutyric acid – has a role in reducing neuron activity in the brain and central nervous system; the benefits include its function in boosting sleep. Like melatonin, it can also be taken as a supplement. It has been described by Dr Michael J Breus as "the brakes of the brain" as it is effectively a catalyst to moving us into a lower gear.[3]

Linked to its benefits in reducing stress and anxiety, GABA can help us both relax and fall asleep, then stay asleep. Conversely, low GABA activity is linked to insomnia and disrupted sleep.[4]

Research has confirmed that exercise has a positive effect on the quality of sleep. A study of different groups of participants reported that those who exercised regularly slept longer than those who did not. In evaluating the effect of an exercise programme on various obstructive sleep apnoea (OSA) indices, it has also been found that exercise is pretty much the only thing associated with improved sleep outcomes in adult. So, you've got no excuse now – get exercising![5]

It's good to know that there is multiple research to back the positive connection between exercise and sleep. In a 2014 study at the University of Georgia, the lead author, Richard Dishman, having found a positive correlation between fitness and sleep, says, "Staying active won't cure sleep complaints ... but it will reduce the odds of them."[6] A study from Bellarmine University and Oregon State University confirmed that, "regular physical activity (of 150 minutes per week) may serve as a non-pharmaceutical alternative to improve sleep."[7] A University of Pennsylvania study showed that those who walked regularly slept better. And lead author, Michael Grandner, confirmed, "these effects are even stronger for more purposeful activities, such as running and yoga, and even gardening and golf."[8]

However, don't expect an overnight difference. A 2013 study from Northwestern University suggested that regular exercise added 45 minutes sleep to your night; however, the full benefits could take four months to be felt.[9]

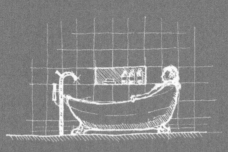

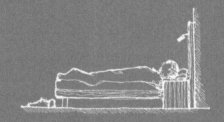

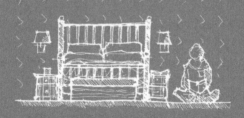

PART FOUR

SLEEP WELLBEING

CHAPTER 20:
MORE SLEEP
COULD IMPACT YOUR
PERFORMANCE

Before our mid-30s we often tend to think that we can cut corners on sleep. Much of the earlier chapters have illustrated the long-term and short-term damage of this. Here I will focus more on some of the benefits that better sleep can bring. I will draw from a couple of distinct angles to demonstrate the key points, one for people in organizations and the other in the world of sport, where being in peak physical and mental shape can be the difference between winning and losing.

A great source of research on sleep and its relationship to work – and especially leadership – is the work of Nick van Dam and Els van der Helm. Their study[1] is an excellent reminder – based on hard data from a closed survey of 200 business leaders. Despite the fact that tired leaders often make irrational claims such as 'I do not need sleep' and 'I'm doing fine with a couple of hours,' the survey suggested that more than half the leaders were dissatisfied with the quality (55%) and quantity (66%) of their sleep, many putting the blame at their organization's door.

The functioning of a key part of the brain for getting things done – the prefrontal cortex – is strongly affected by how much sleep we get. This may sound a bit complex; however, stick with me and I'll do my best to explain.

It seems widely accepted that the last part of our brain to evolve is the neocortex. This area is responsible for functions like language, for planning and executing voluntary movements and for sensory perception. The front part of the neocortex is, in turn, called the prefrontal cortex, which directs our so-called 'executive functions'. As mentioned above, this covers many processes that help us to get things done – problem-solving, reasoning, organization, planning and carrying out those plans.

Now look at that list and you can see that key leadership behaviours rely on at least one of these processes, and hence on the prefrontal cortex in particular. Neuroscientists have observed that while visual and motor skills deteriorate in people who lack sleep, it's nothing compared to the effect of sleep deprivation on what van der Helm and van Dam call 'higher order mental skills.'[2] And the good news is that, as you might have guessed, the reverse can be said to be true. Sleep in the right quantity and quality can boost your ability to perform these so-called executive functions.

Four key positive qualities supported by good sleep worth highlighting are:

THE BENEFITS OF GOOD SLEEP FOR LEADERS

RESULTS ORIENTATION

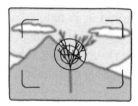

SOLVING PROBLEMS EFFECTIVELY

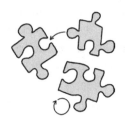

SEEKING DIFFERENT PERSPECTIVES

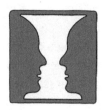

SUPPORTING OTHERS

1. **Results orientation** – Critically linked to attention and concentration, this is the ability to stay focused and see the bigger picture. Scientists have shown that after being awake for 20 hours an individual's performance equals that of someone with a blood-alcohol level of 0.1%, the precise definition of being drunk (in the US).[3] So, to stay focused and keep perspective on the wider issues, a good night's sleep on a regular basis is a wonderful start.

2. **Solving problems effectively** – The mental capacities supporting this, and strongly affected by sleep, are creativity, development of insight and pattern recognition. Studies have shown that a good night's sleep can help you spot shortcuts to solving problems, and an afternoon nap taken before 3pm has similar properties. And, of course, REM sleep has great creative thinking properties, allowing for the integration of information to develop creative solutions.

3. **Seeking different perspectives** – This definitely goes out of the window when you are tired! After all, why would you want to listen to another person's viewpoint late in the day if you have an idea what to do and simply want to get away from the office? The mental capacities of learning (and willingness to learn), memory and decision-making all require good quality and quantity of sleep to enable you to seek different perspectives. As van der Helm and van Dam put it, multiple scientific studies highlight "... the impact of sleep on all three stages of the learning process – before learning, to encode new information; after learning, in the consolidation stage, when the brain forms new connections; and before remembering, to retrieve information from memory."[4] Weighing up options, plus avoiding tunnel vision and bias, help a leader seek different perspectives. And, in order to avoid making critical decisions when tired, 'sleeping on it' is well advised.

4. **Supporting others** – Lastly, emotional reactions and developing trusted relationships, which both benefit from a good night's sleep, are key to a person's ability to support the teams they lead and those they work with. That's because to help others you must first have some level of understanding of them. Often this comprehension is best achieved through non-verbal cues; in other words, it's not 'what' they say but 'how' they say it via

their facial expression or tone of voice. Research suggests that when sleep deprived, we are more likely to misread these cues, to overreact and to be more negative. Other studies show we trust less when sleep deprived, and even that our teams will be less engaged when we are in this state.

Clearly the above qualities – when enhanced and sustained through good sleep – show up in the world of sport too. However, the acknowledgment of sleep as a significant – perhaps even ultimate – performance enhancer in sport is certainly a phenomenon from the last 50 years. As a childhood sports fan and player I recall any game being all about victory and defeat, great heroes who had performed superhuman efforts to win, and gallant, sportsmanlike losers. Sport is still that today, with the addition of much more talk of the 'inner game' and nutrition. And of recovery – a key element in both competing and training – to enable you to come back stronger.

Half a century ago, talk of the need for regeneration would have set most of us thinking about *Star Trek*. Today, it's a common topic for any serious athlete with sleep at the heart of an effective strategy. Muscle, tissue and dead cells are all renewed and replaced during sleep. In fact, based on this, there seems to be some irrefutable logic to say that the harder you train, the more sleep you will need.

Roger Federer is an example of a sporting legend who values his sleep. Not many of us can do as Federer allegedly did, which is rent two houses next door to each other before and during Wimbledon in case he needed to escape the noise of the family for a decent night's rest. However, there are some interesting lessons from the world of sport that we can take into other areas of life. Here are five:[5]

THE BENEFITS OF GOOD SLEEP TO ATHLETES

FASTER REACTIONS

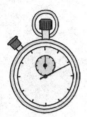

ENHANCED ACCURACY

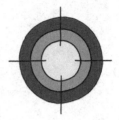

REDUCED INJURY

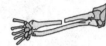

FEWER ERRORS

$$112 \div 4 = ?$$

LONGER CAREERS

1. **Improved reaction time:** We already know that going for 20 hours without sleep is the equivalent of being drunk. Research shows that properly rested people, getting an average of 7.5 hours of sleep a day, can have 2–3 times the reaction times of those who are sleep deprived.[6] A vital advantage in sport, and a useful one in the daily lives of those of us who drive, debate or do anything that needs a quick response.

A good night's sleep on a regular basis is a wonderful start.

2. **Reduced injury rate and improvement in overall health:** Multiple studies point to this, including one from the University of California showing that injury rates in young athletes climb as soon as they sleep less than six hours a night. In other research it was found that the amount of sleep a high school athlete had was the strongest predictor of injuries, more accurate than the number of hours of practice or indeed any other parameter.[7]

   This is because fatigue affects your reaction time and can, in turn, increase the likelihood of injuries. In addition, poor sleep harms our immune system, making us more susceptible to illness. And, finally, shorter overall sleep periods fail to provide the body with time to regenerate cells, muscle and tissue. Merely a more extreme example of something that is true for us all.

3. **Longer playing careers:** If the Roger Federer example isn't enough to convince you, some research into Major League Baseball might. The latter suggests an almost linear correlation between plenty of sleep to performance and career length.[8] Now, that's worth a lot to most people, especially when their cognitive or physical skills are vital in performing a role.

4. **Better accuracy and faster sprint times:** This has been observed in basketball, swimming and tennis, among other sports. And surely, it's no coincidence that cheetahs – among the fastest animals on the planet travelling from zero to 60 mph in three seconds – routinely sleep up to 18 hours per day.

5. **Fewer mental errors:** Vital for sportsmen and women, plus, at the very least, very helpful to the rest of us in multiple ways.

So, we can see why sleep and its benefits have become a competitive edge in sport. As one professional triathlete, Jarrod Shoemaker, puts it, "Sleep is half my training."

Another positive contribution to the sleep debate stemming from the world of sport is Nick Littlehales' R90 method. Using a constant morning wake-up time as the anchor of his recommendation, Littlehales suggests that we think of sleep as 90-minute cycles, with the optimum night's sleep equaling five complete cycles per day (as shown in the graph in Chapter 11), or 35 cycles per week. Littlehales has become well known for his work in 'programming sleep' for British Cycling, Premiership football and rugby sides, plus Olympic and Paralympic teams.

Using this method, we can calculate the optimum time to sleep and wake up. If you need to get up at 6.30am every day, it would be beneficial to aim to go to sleep at 11pm. Interestingly though, Littlehales is such a strong advocate of sleeping full 90-minute cycles (and hence avoiding alarm clocks where possible), that he recommends that if you miss that 11pm bedtime, go to bed at 12.30am instead and stick to a 6.30am wake-up. This is based on his belief that sleeping a multiple of full sleep cycles is best, and hence recommends you sleep from 11pm to 6.30am (five cycles), for example, or 12.30am to 6.30am (four cycles). If you sleep four cycles, Littlehales' recommendation is that you catch up with a 90 minute nap (one sleep cycle) later in the day.

He also advocates aiming for four nights a week of five full sleep cycles, and an overall minimum of 28 cycles per week.[9] Littlehales is also a strong advocate of 'bookending' your day with pre- and post-sleep periods of calm that help you let the old day out and welcome in a new one. More of this to come.

The Harvard Medical School has propagated the idea of sleep being one of three key pillars of health, along with diet and exercise. In fact, I agree with Matthew Walker when I say that for me sleep is now the foundation of my health, with diet and exercise being additional pillars built upon the sleep foundation. Get the foundation wrong and the other two won't help you nearly as much as they would if you were sleeping optimally.

For the majority, they are part of some sort of organization – be it for work, education or something else. So, in looking at sleep wellbeing as an overall topic I will start with what organizations can do, before moving on to individual sleep wellbeing.

THE FOUNDATIONS OF HEALTH AND WELLBEING

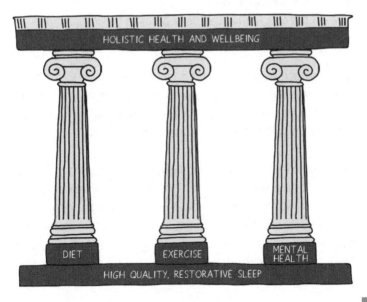

HOLISTIC HEALTH AND WELLBEING

DIET   EXERCISE   MENTAL HEALTH

HIGH QUALITY, RESTORATIVE SLEEP

CHAPTER 21: WHAT CAN ORGANIZATIONS DO TO PROMOTE BETTER SLEEP?

To make sense of the myriad options open to organizations here – and there is genuinely quite a range – I will categorize the choices into three main areas:

- What the leader can do.
- What the organization can do to promote the right culture.
- What organizations can do to target sleep specifically.

This approach is not meant to be 'mutually exclusive,' so there may well be overlaps between categories. It is also not meant to be a completely exhaustive list, but merely one that you, the reader, can use as a prompt to stimulate discussion and hopefully expand upon.

Let's start with the leader. Whether you are a CEO with 100,000 employees, the owner of a small business, or whatever type of leader, the way you behave, and in this case the habits you form around sleep, are incredibly important in shaping the way the organization will evolve on this topic. Reading Arianna Huffington's *The Sleep Revolution* reminded me that we have made some progress since George Costanza – a character in the TV show *Seinfeld* who built a custom bed-desk in his office to keep his napping habit a secret. However, so many of us appear to be defined by our work. So many people end up putting work first and making everything else fit around it. Moving back to a 'human being' from a 'human doing' is easier said than done; however, the role of the leader is to inspire this critical change.

Apart from Huffington's own experience of burnout that led her to wake up on the floor of the CNN studios in a pool of blood, having collapsed from exhaustion, she cites many high-profile examples of different actions to inspire a culture where sleep matters. For me the most useful and practical is that of Karen May, Google's vice president of people development, who realized that she was not making the tough choices she needed to, and hence was putting work – and saying yes – before sleep. This is a description of her practical and instructive tips to overcome this:

- Focus on quantity – if you are not in bed you cannot sleep, so focus on getting to bed earlier and earlier over time.
- Focus on quality – monitor what you eat and drink from 2pm onwards (including cutting out coffee after lunch) and doing something last thing at night other than work, such as sudoku or a crossword puzzle.
- Be accountable – check-in with your partner or a buddy who you've agreed to be completely honest with about your sleep and see how they can help.
- Play the long game – it's the little incremental changes that add up.

Let's examine some of the practical steps a leader can take that can prove visible within the organization.[1]

1. When possible, do not schedule meetings before 9am or after 6pm. Be mindful of the time zones of others and ask yourself if those global telephone calls truly have to be global or if you cannot do them by geographical regions sometimes and play back – perhaps literally! – input from others. When I was based in London, running a global team almost 20 years ago, I can recall hearing a colleague from Melbourne snoring on the other end of the line, then waking up rather noisily and hanging up. What was the point of that?

2. Set boundaries on times that emails can be sent. For example, do not reply to emails after 9pm (6pm on a Friday) and before 7am the next day and not on weekends. This will help everyone get some rest. Every rule has its exceptions – such as it being a matter of life and death, losing a customer or the factory burning down. Unless you've promised a 24/5 service and have another one or two peers situated in other time zones to do your job (assume trading houses do), then you are entitled to some rest that will enable you to regenerate and come back refreshed the next day. Limit access to work emails during off-work hours and weekends.

3. Talking of traders, one way they often limit the time of meetings is having standing meetings. This helps people focus on the really important stuff. A daily standing check-in of 15 minutes to talk about what's critical can be very efficient and enable you to get home earlier.

4. Being open about your need for rest/sleep/switching off is a strength. Just like leaving early to pick up the kids from school on a regular afternoon every week, or taking a proper break for lunch. Setting this example matters. If you make it clear to your team that after 16 hours awake – hopefully not all of it at work – you need some sleep, it will have an impact.

5. When the weather allows it, encourage walking meetings. I now do this with my coaching clients when the weather allows. I take a pocket notebook with me to scribble any key take outs down I don't think I'll be able to remember. Providing the weather is favourable, these 'wisdom walks' will often produce a better outcome than being seated at a table.

And here are a few additional tips on sleep and travel based on some advice from Els van der Helm. These are great for a leader to role model, an organization to encourage and even embed in policy where possible, and for individuals to choose to adopt:

- Be mindful when picking flights – avoiding 'red eyes' plus early-morning and late-night flights where at all possible.
- Booking the same hotel chain, even the same room where possible, when you visit somewhere regularly, helps to start to make it feel like home. Even better if it is a walking distance to where you are working so you may have the opportunity to get some fresh air and daylight exposure.
- Pack things you need to help your sleep routine, e.g. an eye mask, your own wake-up light alarm clock (not the same as your phone), etc.

- Many hotels do have formally designated quiet bedrooms. If not, reservations will often know which ones are quieter. Ask for one of these to give yourself the best chance of sleep.
- Keep the room at about 19°C for sleep and if you don't have blackout curtains, ask for clips or bring pegs to make sure the room is dark.
- Work in the lounge when you need to. The more you can associate the hotel bedroom with sleep the better.
- Look to keep other things as similar as possible to home, keeping in touch with friends and family, eating sensibly and continuing to exercise.

From an organizational perspective, there is plenty that can be done to support leaders, teams and individuals. Increasingly, there is a recognition that more and better quality sleep makes us better at our jobs, which typically then reminds us that we are more than simply what we do for work.

Given the opportunity for this virtuous circle to exist, and also that work seems to be the number one cause of people missing out on sleep, here are some examples for developing a positive work culture that may promote positive sleep:

- **Flexible working arrangements:** These are now more common and studies indicate that greater autonomy in how people schedule their time does help employees sleep more. This makes sense as it enables night owls to sleep later and start work later, or to work from home and use the commuting time saved to finish earlier, exercise, pick the kids up from school or simply sleep more. Research also suggests that productivity can improve at home with fewer distractions, plus people that are able to work more at their own rhythm and at the best times of the day get less distracted and have the opportunity to nap.

- **Office windows and natural light:** Another fascinating study suggests that employees in offices with windows get three quarters of an hour more sleep per night than those that don't have the same access to natural light. According to the study author, Dr Phyllis Zee:[2] "There is increasing evidence that exposure to light during the day – particularly in the morning – is beneficial to your health via its effects on mood, alertness and metabolism."

- **Smart technology:** Utilize smart technology such as applications to reduce the blue light on computers that can inhibit the production of the sleep hormone, melatonin.

- **Nap rooms:** Arianna Huffington, now something of a sleep guru herself, admits to being sceptical about nap rooms being placed in her company's New York offices in 2011. After a slow initial take up, they are now well used, with other companies like Nike and Ben & Jerry's taking a similar approach.

- **Technology:** This is so often blamed for promoting a 24/7 work culture that is harmful to sleep. However, it can be harnessed for the benefit of creating a culture that encourages sleep. The example I hear quoted most often is that the car maker Volkswagen turns off company email servers half an hour after the official end of the working day. Other German companies, such as BMW and Deutsche Telekom, are following suit. And in France an agreement between the employers' federations and unions allows employees in certain sectors to turn off their phones after work.

Make it clear to your team that after 16 hours awake – hopefully not all of it at work – you need some sleep.

Many of the above are harder to incorporate than simply training staff about good sleep practice. In the same way I had to take a time management course as a graduate trainee in the mid-1980s, it would be great, nowadays, to also have sleep management being taught. Technology can be used to support this.

And for a more radical approach, your organization can choose to adopt unilaterally to follow the lead of the US software company that gives employees a US$7,500 bonus if they follow two rules: (1) They have to actually go on vacation or they don't get the money; (2) They must disconnect, and hence cannot work, on vacation.

An additional radical yet practical example was shared in 2019 by the World Economic Forum.[3] "A Japanese Company is paying its staff to sleep more. To make sure they are well-rested, productive and happy at work, Tokyo-based Crazy Inc. is offering 'points' to workers who sleep at least six hours a night at least five days a week. The points can be exchanged in the company cafeteria. And they are worth up to US$570 per year to those who get the most sleep. The company tracks sleep data via an app. The project aims to solve a range of health problems associated with a lack of sleep." The post goes on to suggest the Rand Corporation estimates that the Japanese economy loses US$138 billion a year due to sleep-related health problems, and the United States $411 billion based on the same analysis.

And while I recommend putting the smartphones and electronic tablets away as a route to better sleep, I can certainly see the point of apps like f.lux, which limit blue light on these devices, in addition to the technology to help alleviate jet lag mentioned earlier.

Huffington adds her own sleep wish list.[4] Here are four of my favourites that I think could come about one day:

- Nap mats become as commonplace as yoga mats at work.
- A public-awareness campaign for drowsy driving comparable to the one against drunk driving is launched.
- Education about the dangers of drowsy driving is added to the warnings against drunk driving in drivers' education classes.
- A test for drowsiness is developed – similar to the breathalyzer – so that drowsy driving can be measured and regulated.

CHAPTER 22: WHAT CAN INDIVIDUALS DO FOR BETTER SLEEP?

Have you ever fallen asleep in a meeting? Go on, admit it ... Well, I have loads of times. In the past, you understand – I'm pleased to say I haven't done so for a while. However, have you ever fallen asleep in a one-to-one meeting? Well, unfortunately, after a big night out in my misspent youth, I have to plead guilty to that one. And what about while interviewing someone for a job? Surely that's the most embarrassing and least professional of the lot!

It was 1999 and I was ending a long-term assignment in Vietnam. I had been interviewing in Hanoi all the previous week – up to eight one-hour slots – a handful of excellent candidates and 50 that ranged from, at best, pretty average to, at worst, fairly hopeless. That was only half the story, however. My interviewing partner was our HR director. And I was struggling to take her seriously as her three questions were always the same: (1) What are your strengths and weaknesses? (2) Where do you see yourself in five years' time and (3) ... to be honest, I forget!

I was predominantly based in Ho Chi Minh City in the south of Vietnam, so I decided to spread this work trip to Hanoi over two weeks and take a weekend trip with some friends to Sapa, a fascinating area on the Chinese border. So, after taking a night train on Friday and another on Sunday night, I was pretty short of sleep by 3pm Monday afternoon. When – in my opinion – our worst candidate yet appeared. And I nodded off.

I cannot recall how I woke up; however, when I did the candidate was staring at me and proceeded to give me a piece of his mind. And then my colleague the HR director followed. I was sorely tempted to retort that it was her questioning technique that had driven me to taking a nap, but I resisted. So, unless you have access to sleeping pods at work or a George Costanza contraption, you will need to develop good sleeping habits that will serve you personally and professionally. Here are some suggestions to help you sleep better:

- **Avoid all forms of sleeping pill medication:** This will not help you in a sustainable way unless you want to be taking them for life. Don't start. There is also substantial evidence to suggest that when you stop taking them, you'll initially have worse sleeping problems than when you started. It simply isn't worth it. Sometimes termed 'rebound insomnia,' this comes from a patient developing a certain tolerance of the drug, because that's what a sleeping pill is – a drug. However, like any drug, when the sleeping pills are removed, the user suffers withdrawal, and this often leads to even worse insomnia than the patient had before taking the pills.
- **Use of melatonin:** Some say the use of melatonin is a form of taking medication. I would personally see it as more of a natural supplement. It seems effective in some cases; however, one of the challenges with melatonin is that it's unregulated

and hence no two brands of melatonin have the same percentage melatonin content. If you find a brand that works for you, I suggest that you stick to it. Don't assume another product will perform as well. The other thing – as mentioned in the section on circadian rhythm sleep disorders – is taking the melatonin at the same time daily so it works in the same way with the circadian cycle and the sleep pressure that builds up every day.

- **Cognitive Behavioural Therapy (CBT):** This is strongly advocated by some of the respected writers I've read, and it may work for some. However, I am much more persuaded by my own experiences, plus the arguments of Dr Guy Meadows, the founder of the Sleep School.[1] As he points out, CBT unhelpfully focuses on trying to get rid of the symptoms associated with poor sleep. Hence, your energy is focused on what you don't want rather than on what you do want, which is to sleep. My belief – based on my personal experience – is that a more holistic approach involving a better diet and more exercise is a more sustainable solution in the long term. However, there are plenty of respected sources that advocate CBT.

- **Regular routine:** There is much to be said for having a regular routine. Even Nick Littlehales' revolutionary R90 theory – which challenges lots of orthodoxies about sleep such as the need for eight hours per night – advocates a constant waking up time as its anchor. Of course, it's sensible to aim to align and respect our natural circadian rhythm.

- **Sleep hygiene:** This is another area that gets a lot of attention and, again, while I don't believe it was critical to the improvement in my own sleep, there is certainly a case for having as good a bed and mattress as you can afford, having the room temperature circa 19°C (or whatever works for you), using blackout curtains/blinds or similar and using a wake-up light alarm clock if you need one at all. Having said all that, I have to say that the adverts running on the London Underground seem so memorable I want to rush out and try the product. "We have drift off!" they proclaim. "The world's first height adjustable pillow made with temperature regulating technology designed for astronauts." "Time to space out," say the posters from SIMBA. Their parallel mattress ads are headlined, "The unrest is history."

- **Other recommendations:** Specifically for those suffering from obstructive sleep apnoea (OSA), I would recommend the use of a continuous positive airway pressure (CPAP) machine. It takes getting used to; however, it's helped my sleep quality a lot and it's available on the NHS. Hooray! Otherwise machines seem to vary from as little as £100 to in excess of £2,000, depending on size and portability.

CHAPTER 23:
HOW TO SLEEP
BETTER: TOP 10
PERSONAL TIPS
– 'BOOKENDING YOUR NIGHT'

Whenever I give talks about sleep, primarily to business leaders, I'm always asked for my top tips. So, here they are – a personal list of what's worked best for me, my top 10 tips to aid good sleep. The first four are general good lifestyle practices that – put simply – support sleep. Numbers five to ten are ideas of how to 'bookend your night.' I trust they will be of use to you.

1. **Carefully manage (or quit) the caffeine!** I was a 'seven espressos' a day man when I quit in 2015. I had an espresso machine by my office desk and one at home. I would justify the one in the office with a story about signing a deal when I was managing director of a business in Papua New Guinea (PNG). The purchasing director from our largest customer – a gold mine that accounted for more than 20% of PNG's GDP at the time – was coming to see me in my office to sign – or otherwise – a contract extension worth USD 100 million per year in revenues. Kyle (not his real name) was pretty bullish on the phone – said he only had an hour to sort this deal out, which we'd been discussing for months. So, there were a few nervous people in my office.

When Kyle appeared I offered him an espresso. He seemed immediately impressed. The meeting flowed well. We were prepared and rapport was good. After 30 minutes Kyle said, "Can I have another one of those wonderful espressos?" The contract was signed 43 minutes later, with no alterations.

Clearly, I was an addict, using stories like the one above to justify my habit like any addict would. However, even if you are not a 'coffee junkie' like I was, treating caffeine after lunch as a no-no – except in extreme circumstances – can only help your sleep.

2. **Do a thorough diet detox twice a year and learn to eat clean(er).**
    This is linked to #1 in that when I detox I give up caffeine (which in my case would only be in dark chocolate or the occasional green tea), alcohol, dairy products plus carbohydrates. The detox process I follow lasts three weeks and the benefits are multiple – weight loss, more energy, better hair (well it certainly grows faster!), improved skin and even better sleep. This is linked to the diet observations made earlier and aims to create the best conditions for sleep-enhancing hormones like dopamine and GABA to flourish.

3. **Exercise:** Intuitively, it makes sense you'll sleep better if you exercise regularly. Some form of sport, or even a brisk walk in the day, will typically leave you feeling more tired. My personal tip is, if possible, fit walking into your commute. From spring to autumn I typically walk three tube stops through the park to work as one way to squeeze in exercise in a busy schedule. Also I've always been a morning exerciser out of preference, which means that the adrenaline and other hormones released when you physically exert yourself get a chance to work their way through the system before turning in for the night.

I find tracking my exercise endeavours on a smartphone app of some sort gives a sense of satisfaction and achievement. Personally, I use the sports tracker Strava, though there are many on offer.

4. **Naps:** These are a great way to get quality sleep during the day, but with two main caveats. First, whenever you take them, do wake up before 3pm so that you do not disrupt your night sleep too much. Second, try to take naps of circa 26 minutes (as recommended by NASA) or circa 90 minutes (the full sleep cycle) in length. This way you are much less likely to wake up feeling 'groggy.'

For those yet to experience the joys and benefits of napping, whether you feel guilty about doing so or remain sceptical, Arianna Huffington has surveyed a myriad of research and literature to help understand why naps are so restorative. She quotes David Randall, the author of *Dreamland*, as saying that even a short nap "primes our brains to function at a higher level, letting us come up with better ideas, find solutions to puzzles more quickly, identifying patterns faster and recall information more accurately."

Like Huffington, I used the couch in my office when I was managing director of a business in Sri Lanka. However, unlike her I did not have the courage to remove the screen on the window of my office door so that people could see what I was doing. Perhaps if I'd known this quote from Winston Churchill then it would have inspired me. Let's leave the last word on naps to him: "You must sleep sometime between lunch and dinner, and no half measures. Take off your clothes and get into bed.

That's what I always do. Don't think you will be doing less work because you sleep during the day. That's a foolish notion held by people who have no imaginations. You will be able to accomplish more. You get two days in one – well, at least one and a half."[1]

BOOKENDING YOUR NIGHT

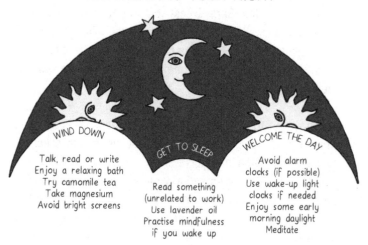

WIND DOWN
Talk, read or write
Enjoy a relaxing bath
Try camomile tea
Take magnesium
Avoid bright screens

GET TO SLEEP
Read something
(unrelated to work)
Use lavender oil
Practise mindfulness
if you wake up

WELCOME THE DAY
Avoid alarm
clocks (if possible)
Use wake-up light
clocks if needed
Enjoy some early
morning daylight
Meditate

Another important idea is to 'bookend your night.' This is a simple concept that seeks to build on existing literature to give you some easy to follow guidelines:

- Let the old day out – unwind properly and give yourself the best chance of sleep (#5,#6 and also #8)
- Sleep – what to do if you wake up in the night and struggle to go back to sleep (#7 and #8)
- Let the new day in – allowing your day to start calmly before overtaken by events and the agenda of others (#9 and 10)

5. Give yourself enough time to wind down: Allow the experiences of the day to come out of your mind. Read, talk, make love, and don't look at a smartphone – all great ways to let the old day out. It is also something that is more in your control. Nick Littlehales is adamant that 90 minutes to unwind plus another 90 minutes to wind up again in the morning is ideal, and he may well be right.[2] However, from my experience even one hour to bookend your day can make a huge difference.

Start by turning off smartphones, tablets, computers and, preferably, TVs too. A daily technology detox of circa 11 hours is an ideal – 90 minutes before bedtime, 8 hours for sleep and 90 minutes once you wake up. Sound a bit too radical? Well aiming for 9.5 hours (1 hour letting the day out + 7.5 hours of sleep + 1 hour letting the day in) would be a great start.

Other ways to 'declutter the mind' before you go sleep include tidying up, doing the dishes or putting the washing on, writing a journal or scribbling down some thoughts on what's on your mind – all good ways to prepare for sleep.

And if you want to read before you sleep, do read paper – a book or a magazine for example.

I have always found chamomile tea or something similar is a great help. Whether or not this is a reaction akin to that of a Pavlovian dog I cannot say, though a cursory google of 'chamomile tea' and 'sleep' suggests there is some science behind this. And another advantage of chamomile tea is that it tastes great cold so you can enjoy it if you wake in the middle of the night.

6. **Epsom salt baths:** A wonderful relaxant, magnesium being the key ingredient. Indeed there appears to be a medical consensus that the population of many developing countries are magnesium deficient. As this essential mineral is not produced within our own bodies, we effectively need to import it. Magnesium is more easily absorbed through the skin rather than orally and a bath is a great way to access an incremental boost to aid your sleep.

Magnesium deficiency can manifest itself in insomnia. Conversely, appropriate levels of magnesium support deep, restorative sleep through maintaining GABA levels, the neurotransmitter mentioned earlier that promotes sleep. Magnesium is also supposed to help alleviate restless legs syndrome, which is sometimes linked to insomnia.[3]

Please note: Epsom salts are to be avoided if you have open wounds or sores. Also they have been known to cause irritation if you have very sensitive skin. In this case a magnesium rich diet, including sunflower seeds, cashew nuts and almonds plus squash and broccoli, can be helpful.

In addition to – or as an alternative to – an Epsom salt bath, use lavender oil close to you when you sleep. Place one or two drops on a cotton pad or tissue/handkerchief on your bedside table (preferably on a saucer to prevent any oil stains). Add one or two drops more if you want a stronger dose. Some people prefer to place this on a tissue under their pillow. Whichever approach you take should yield positive results.

7. **Use mindfulness techniques:** For example, use body scanning if you wake in the night. I mentioned body scanning earlier, also known as 'noticing sensations and urges,' a technique whereby you start with your toes and slowly scan up through your whole body until you reach the top of your head, stopping along the way to bring an awareness to each part of your body. I find this especially helpful in addressing the 3am syndrome.

If you especially like mindfulness techniques, I urge you to read *The Sleep Book: How to Sleep Well Every Night* by Dr Guy Meadows,[4] which has many similar suggestions.

8. **Read in bed:** A book, newspaper or magazine not related to your work is a fantastic way to relax. I believe that technically Kindles are fine too; however, I've always favoured making that complete break from technology to allow you to do something different in a different medium. I read an entire biography of P.G. Wodehouse between 3 and 4am once which helped me get back to sleep every time. Sudoku helps many people in the same way. And once again, unlike smartphones, tablets, computers and the TV, paper seems less likely to increase our stress and alertness.

9. **Avoid alarm clocks where you can:** Why is this? Well it will give you the best chance of waking up naturally at the end of a sleep cycle, and mitigate any grogginess which can sometimes happen. And if you absolutely must set one because you are catching a flight or something similar, do not set multiple alarms for the morning as this will only encourage snoozing. If you need one, use a wake-up light alarm clock.

10. Meditate in the morning to let the day in: The simplest way to do this is to sit upright or in the cross-legged position (whichever is more natural for you) with a hand on each knee or with hands resting upwards in your lap. Close your eyes and breathe in through your nose for a count of two, hold for two and then out for four. Breathe in through the stomach as much as possible (much as babies do), avoiding short breaths in the chest. Manage this basic technique based on yoga teachings for five minutes a day and it will set you on the road to deeper meditation.

Ultimately, a lot of this comes down to individual choice. Prioritize your health and wellbeing, and within that sleep as the foundation.

A footnote on technology: You may have noticed the almost complete absence of technology in these top 10 tips, largely because most apps that can support sleep are accessed via personal smartphones or tablets, which may also prompt the user to look at emails and other messages. This is highly likely to 'wind up' the brain rather than allow it to wind down. However, there are apps that can help you track your sleep progress over time and prompt you to try different techniques to improve it. I have developed an online sleep course with Nikki Owen and will shortly launch this. Please email me directly via Giles@Positivesleep.co.uk, should you want to know more.

Don't think you will be doing less work because you sleep during the day. That's a foolish notion held by people who have no imaginations.

Winston Churchill

And for those who value measurement as part of their self-diagnosis I recommend a couple of options:

- If you wish to gauge your degree of sleep fulfilment please fill in the five questions comprising the SATED questionnaire at **https://www.ncbi.nlm.nih.gov**[5]

- And to check out the likelihood of you suffering from sleep apnoea it's worth measuring yourself on the Epworth Sleepiness Scale (ESS). The associated survey is available from multiple sources including **https://britishsnoring.co.uk**

CHAPTER 24:
THE FUTURE OF
SLEEP PART ONE –
TECHNOLOGY

Since the first edition of this book, the evolution of technology, especially Artificial Intelligence (AI) has been extraordinary. Hence I wanted to reflect on this and offer up some observations on how this might affect sleep.

At this point I must offer up a caveat: I have been something of a 'technophobe' from a young age. I can only put this down to coming from a wonderful, talented family with a father who was a Chartered Instrument and Mechanical Engineer and an older brother who grew up to be a Rocket Scientist! My sense is that – surrounded by such intense interest in science and technology – I would either grow up to embrace this or run the other way. And I – sadly – ran the other way! However, one thing I did gain from this was an awareness that the application of science and technology was vitally important and was continually life changing to many. Another good reason for the existence of this chapter.

I am also fortunate that I now live very close to the University of Bristol (UoB), where I studied undergraduate Economics 40 years ago. One of many changes at the UoB has been the establishment of a four-year integrated Master's Innovation Programmes within the last decade, which seeks to promote a:

"... collaborative approach which allows students to draw on their subject specialism while collaborating in multidisciplinary teams to deliver new and innovative solutions to a real world challenges."[1] Hence, students develop skills in areas like problem-solving and project management whilst still studying more traditional disciplines.[2]

So, given the changes in technology & the opportunities and threats they represent to sleep, I thought it would great to brief some of the students to examine: ***"How might we use technology to help people sleep better, both now and in the future?"***[3] I was able to get three groups of diverse second-year undergraduates – mostly in their late teens or early 20s – to address this question. Here is what the teams, named Team Ten, Team Three and Team Twelve, came up with:

All three teams were guided in their initial research by Dan Nessler's (2016) 'Revamped Double Diamond' framework. As the team that Team Ten put it, "This split our project into two distinct 'diamonds' – 'Designing the right thing' and 'Designing things right' – each containing four phases – Research, Synthesis, Ideation, and Implementation (Metcalfe, 2016). This strategic model helped us define our problem precisely, leading us to ask the right questions and providing the steps involved in coming up with a solution that could be pitched."[4] All groups engaged in desk-based research, had at least two sessions with me to help them develop their ideas, and liaised with experts in the field, such as Matt Jones, Professor of Neuroscience at the UoB.

Team Three emerged with several practical prototypes that they tested on groups of peers. They included 'the Bluetooth pillow,' which allows a Bluetooth connection between phone and pillow to track sleep and also play music/white noise for a limited time until the user falls asleep. The phone can charge inside the pillow for convenience. A second was named 'the Routine Box,' which charges a phone overnight and incorporates an Alexa (or similar) to track sleep, ask users about their day and their mental state, and try a selection of available methods on the market to help the client sleep, offering multiple solutions. The aim was also that this tool be dynamic, updated regularly with new findings on sleep as information increases.

However, following discussions with potential user groups amongst their peers, the clear winner for Team Three was the lowest tech in many ways: the 'Phone Light Switch' illustrated overleaf. The device is a light switch that holds and charges the user's phone. If the user takes their phone out of the holder, the lights turn on and the phone is returned to its charging point. During the day, you are able to override this with a button and turn the lights on and off as you please. Once you place your phone into the holder, override is not available until the time your alarm is set for. This allows for the lights to function as normal during the day, and then remain off at night for so long.

THE PHONE LIGHT SWITCH

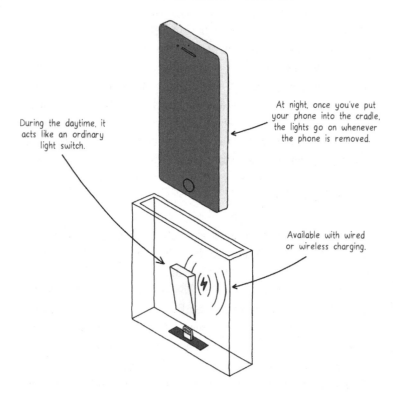

During the daytime, it acts like an ordinary light switch.

At night, once you've put your phone into the cradle, the lights go on whenever the phone is removed.

Available with wired or wireless charging.

The main attribute to this idea is that the user will be discouraged from going on their phone at night because it is out of reach, and going on it would trigger the lights to turn on. This makes the user voluntarily come off their phone and take steps to form a routine, instead of forcing behaviour on them. From the interviews conducted, Team Three found that the majority of people who take steps to put limitations on apps on their phone or set bedtimes end up overriding the restrictions. Hence the idea is that this product will break the habit of going on your phone in bed, and rather prompt you to put the phone in the device. Another function which might be added is a way to turn your lights on to symbolize sunrise just before your alarm is set to go off, much as sunrise alarm clocks do. This creates a more natural wake up and should be easy to combine, as the phone is connected to give alarm data.[5]

Team Ten took an in-depth look at the technology already available as of the first half of 2023. This included:

- 'Wearable and physical sleep aids' such as smart pillows, electromagnetic therapy (e.g. SomniResonance SR1), EEG headbands (e.g. Dreem), electro cranial stimulators (e.g. Fisher Wallace), sleep optimisers (e.g. Sleep Shepherd Blue), headphones and visors (e.g. BrainTap) and sleep-wake lights (e.g. Lumie).
- 'Pharmacological sleep aids' such as medically prescribed sleeping pills, mild tranquilizers and over-the-counter supplements (vitamins, co-enzyme Q10, iron, and magnesium).
- 'Natural sleep aids' such as herbal therapies (valerian root, kava and lavender), pillow sprays, exercise and changes of diet.
- 'Abstract sleep aids' like podcasts and white/pink noise (e.g. Spotify, YouTube), and meditation apps (eg. Headspace).

Having done this, they then undertook primary research to "gain the best understanding of the people we are designing for (the younger demographic)."[6] The team worked with participants from the younger demographic, plus inputs from parents and experts[7] in the field of sleep. Semi-structured interviews, journey maps[8] and cultural probes[9] were used.

Unsurprisingly, their findings were largely supported by Matthew Walker, who found that the majority of young adults experience or present common habits that are widely considered a direct cause of poor sleep including: (i) Neglecting sleep (ii) Oversleeping during the night and/or day to compensate for sleep debt (iii) Overutilizing LED displays and (iv) Lack of self-management.[10]

Through their continuing synthesis and ideation approach, Team One emerged with three ideas. The first was to use my existing website www.positivesleep.co.uk as a portal to a 'customized sleep shop,' stocking affordable products targeting particular sleep problems, such as how to help you get to sleep and how to help you stay asleep. However, ultimately Team One felt that, whilst this shop would be useful, as it allowed consumers to find all the sleeping technologies that one may need in one location, it didn't really cater as much to consumers' bespoke needs, or offer behavioural solutions.

Their second idea was once again to use www.positivesleep.co.uk to offer a free advice section on the most common findings and helpful lifestyle changes to improve sleep hygiene. This condensed snapshot of the most common issues could be attractive to the younger demographic as it is quick and easy to read. Team One's research suggested that focusing on (i) the difficulty of relaxing and getting to sleep, (ii) fatigue after 7-8 hours of sleep, (iii) poor sleep hygiene, (iv) interrupted sleep and (v) sleeping too much would be great starting points. And whilst the merits of this idea included that it offered free advice, which could be easy to implement, it once again was not as tailored a solution to the individual that it would most likely be effective.

Their third idea, which was developed into a prototype, built on the need to 'individualize' sleep programs whilst also making them accessible to everyone. Team One believe that a kind of mass customization approach, whereby arranging the solutions into segments that consist of low cost, low effort, and minimal time commitment, these programs could be individually tailored through an online quiz. The quiz answers would then inform what was offered, tailoring the menu of services made available for a user whilst increasing accessibility.

The final prototype combined the idea of a quiz that could match users to tailored solutions and product suggestions. The prototype web page suggested appropriate sleep technology, help and products prompted by taking a quiz to establish what areas of your sleep needed help, as well as any obstruction to 'Positive Sleep.' Users should be able to sign up via the website and connect their sleep technology to reach more personalised recommendations. Members of the *Positive Sleep* community should also be encouraged (and rewarded) to share and rate their own sleep experiences, as this could help develop an algorithm based on the concept of matching similar lifestyles and common solutions. The data gathered could be refined to produce more tailored sleep recommendations to new users.

POSITIVE SLEEP WEBSITE

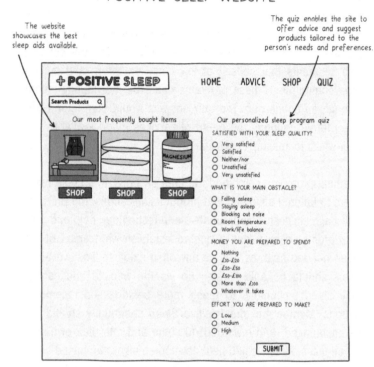

The website showcases the best sleep aids available.

The quiz enables the site to offer advice and suggest products tailored to the person's needs and preferences.

The final group, Team Twelve, blended surveys, interviews and academic paper research to help them gain an understanding of the sleep landscape, where they might help and what prototype they might develop. The team promoted a barcode on campus to get more than 150 students to take their survey, and gained real insights into the sample's sleeping habits, use of technology to help them sleep better (only about 30% had used something), propensity to nap (again only about 1/3 did this), and other issues that this demographic have with sleep. Further expert conversations led Team Twelve to think that educating young adults about the positive effects of good sleep plus the negative impact of poor sleep could be a winner. And after toying with the idea of both a 'Sleep Box' (a lock box for the user's phone to eliminate their ability to look at their screen whilst trying to sleep), and the 'Sleep Bot' (similar to an Alexa, but for sleep, using sounds to create a relaxing environment, control the lighting, ensuring optimality at each stage of the sleep cycle, release soothing aromas, etc. to create a desirable environment), the team settled on the 'Sleep Well' mobile app. This app aims to: "help you fall asleep, learn about sleep and track your sleep habits."[12] A 'learning and earning' focus used non-financial rewards to incentivise use.

MOBILE APP

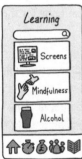
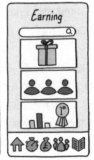
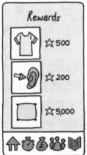

These ideas are all prototypes, and all feel like stepping stones on the way to finding technological solutions to quieten the mind and relax the body. However, there are other ways. Let's explore them.

CHAPTER 25:
THE FUTURE OF
SLEEP PART TWO
- ALTERNATIVE
TECHNOLOGY

Whilst it felt critical to update *Positive Sleep* with some recent trends in digital technology, I was recently prompted to reflect on some ancient wisdom that can also help sleep. As part of my discussion with moderator Mrinali Thalgodapitiya during our session on stage at the Ceylon Literary Festival in Colombo in February, I was asked a number of good questions that clearly linked some more modern techniques to others that have been helping their practitioners to both quieten the mind and relax the body for thousands of years; yoga being a prime example.

It seems to me that many approaches, especially those based on digital technology and/or that focus on data and precise measurement, are actually stressing out the people I talk to about sleep at least as often as these modern tools help them. When using apps and other sleep trackers, many become obsessed with measuring their sleep outcomes and checking them as soon as they wake up. Depending on the results, the user can either be delighted with some material improvement or despondent as they feel their sleep 'went backwards' the previous night.

So it was constructive to hear the views of my friend, Shanaka Amarasinghe – a true polymath – who is an accomplished lawyer, sports commentator, actor and yoga enthusiast (as both a practitioner for 15 years and a teacher for five). Shanka shared some insights from his perspective. "Ultimately sleep is about the two simple – but not easy - tasks of switching off the mind and relaxing the body. It is counterproductive, then, to have these very simple tasks monitored by a smart watch that is interfering with the body's electromagnetic field in the first place. We live in a time where someone who bursts out of bed after three hours feeling as fresh as the proverbial daisy will be devastated by a quick look at their watch, which reminds them they haven't got the requisite number of hours in, putting an immediate damper on their day. Contrast this to the same person who gets a good eight hours in, only to be told that their sleep was sub-optimal because of a multitude of arbitrary data points. The Siege of Data is winning the war on humanity.

"Eastern philosophies – and indeed disciplines/practices – prepare more than just the mind for Life. Practices such as yoga and pranayama have been the refuge of many of us in the Global South for millennia," Shanaka continued. "Giles – one of your favourite techniques of body scanning is, quite literally, the practice of yoga nidra! Indeed, as a yoga practitioner and teacher, I have noticed more and more students hesitant to close their eyes in shavasana (corpse/relaxation pose)."

And how that resonated with me going back to my experience of extreme insomnia, as someone who had been shaken awake long after a yoga class had finished. I found that not only was I the last to leave, but that those waiting outside were laughing at me as I snored blissfully on my back!

Shanaka summed up his thoughts as follows: "Anxiety and fear are the foremost enemies of sleep. One, the other, or both are the reason that yoga students don't trust their environment enough to close their eyes in shavasana. The problem of sleep cannot be solved without solving the problems acquired in wakefulness. It is a 'problem' that can be solved only through the body, as opposed to the mind – that is, if it is a 'problem to be solved' at all.

"Anxiety and fear are states caused in the mind for a multitude of reasons unique to each individual. However, they are felt and stored in the body. Unless we flush them out of the body, they will remain stumbling blocks, not only to sleep, but also to more meaningful waking hours. Your book is the menu outside the restaurant on the tourist strip. If it's promising, you still have to go inside, make an investment and experience the food with your eyes, nose and mouth. Reading your book is a first step in the direction of focusing on one's physical body."

So what's my reflection on this? Well, clearly Shanka reminds us very vividly that quietening the mind goes hand in hand with relaxing the body. This is consistent with 'bookending your night' (p.122) and generally seeing how you wake up and live your day as being instrumental to how well you will sleep at night. However, as a pragmatist rather than a revolutionary, I sense that – at some level – the use of digital technology will remain involved in many people's approach to improving their sleep, especially those born in the 21st century, unless there is some truly dystopian episode which results in a global and permanent digital detox.

And, as for me, it feels like while digital solutions might be useful because they 'speak in the language' that people increasingly adopt these days, I will personally continue to promote 'old tech' solutions. An individual's decisions to shift behaviours to prioritise 'relaxing the body' as well as 'quietening the mind' will – in my opinion – provide the truly committed the greatest chance of harvesting the benefits of *Positive Sleep*.

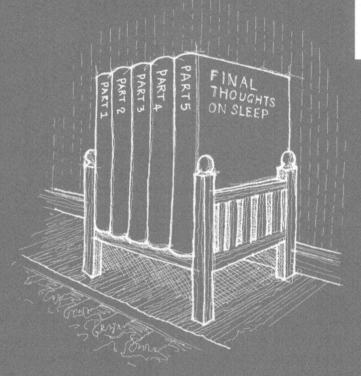

PART FIVE

PART 1
PART 2
PART 3
PART 4
PART 5
FINAL
THOUGHTS
ON SLEEP

FINAL THOUGHTS
ON SLEEP

SUMMARY AND CONCLUSION

Clearly, chronic sleep problems have an impact on an individual's overall wellbeing (personal, social, professional, etc.) across a lifespan. It is important to identify effective treatments and strategies for overcoming sleep problems from a holistic standpoint, incorporating a wide range of perspectives.

Today, there is a discourse on the physiological, cognitive and emotional effects of poor sleep and its complex interactions with one's lifestyle. It had certainly exerted an adverse impact on my daytime functioning and my personal relationships. Furthermore, there is a complex interaction between lifestyle and sleep patterns highlighted by sleep habits and attitudes formed during childhood. These are then carried into and camouflaged during early adulthood, but do not show harm until we are older. The protective mechanism that enables our younger selves to recover from poor sleep patterns begins to decline as we mature.

Effective solutions for sleep issues are often holistic and in-depth. They start from dietary intake and instituting an exercise regimen, as well as incorporating meditation and mindfulness routines to calm the mind.

Proactively addressing professional and personal issues with self-awareness and commitment can help you overcome sleep issues.

FINAL
REFLECTIONS

As well as initiating my journey of recovery from chronic sleep difficulties, writing this book has been highly cathartic in nature. Ultimately, it has forced me to delve deep into myself, which has allowed me to attain greater self-awareness and understanding. This dynamic and iterative approach – having lived the experience I was writing about which, in turn, gave me the impetus to take action and change based on the outcomes I had experienced – has led to a far greater transformation than I could have hoped for or imagined. I have been able to apply the findings to improve the reality of my situation. It has thus offered a powerful validation of the strategies that I had identified as being effective in resolving my chronic sleep problems. As it turned out, the key to resolving them would entail a complete transformation of my life for the better, both from the inside and outside.

My hope for you is that, having read this book, you will be spurred into action if you have sleep issues to address and are now aware of some proven ways to help yourself and others. I wish you every success in your endeavour to benefit from *Positive Sleep*.

REFERENCES

CHAPTER 1

1. Arianna Huffington, *The Sleep Revolution: Transforming Your Life, One Night At A Time* (WH Allen, 2016), p.37

2. Compernolle, T., *BrainChains – Discover your brain and unleash its full potential in a hyperconnected multitasking world* (Amsterdam: Compublications, 2014), p.243

3. van Dam, N. & van der Helm, E., "The organizational cost of insufficient sleep." *McKinsey Quarterly*, 1-9 (February 2016). https://www.mckinsey.com/business-functions/organization/our-insights/the-organizational-cost-of-insufficient-sleep

4. Compernolle, T., *BrainChains – Discover your brain and unleash its full potential in a hyperconnected multitasking world* (Amsterdam: Compublications, 2014)

5. van Dam, N. & van der Helm, E., "The organizational cost of insufficient sleep." *McKinsey Quarterly*, 1-9 (February 2016). https://www.mckinsey.com/business-functions/organization/our-insights/the-organizational-cost-of-insufficient-sleep

6. Goel, N., Rao, H., Durmer, J. S. & Dinges, D. F., "Neurocognitive consequences of sleep deprivation." *Seminars in Neurology*, 29(4), 320–339 (September 2009)

7. Verweij, I. M., Romeijn, N., Smit, D. J. A., Piantoni, G., Van Someren, E.J.W. & van der Werf, Y. D., "Sleep deprivation leads to loss of functional connectivity in frontal brain regions." *BMC Neuroscience, 15* (88) (July 2014). https://bmcneurosci.biomedcentral.com/articles/10.1186/1471-2202-15-88

8. van Dam, N. & van der Helm, E., "The organizational cost of insufficient sleep." *McKinsey Quarterly*, 1-9 (February 2016). https://www.mckinsey.com/business-functions/organization/our-insights/the-organizational-cost-of-insufficient-sleep

CHAPTER 3

1. The Impact Of COVID-19 On Global Sleep Patterns, https://blog.fitbit.com/covid-19-sleep-patterns/

2. Survey Reveals Covid-19 Having Severe Impact on Sleep, https://thesleepcharity.org.uk/survey-reveals-covid-19-having-severe-impact-on-sleep/

3. Sleep Med. Jan 2021; 77: 346–347. Published June 6, 2020. "The acute effects of the COVID-19 pandemic on insomnia and psychological symptoms." Charles M. Morin, Université Laval, Institut Universitaire en Santé Mentale de Québec, Canada, Centre D'étude des Troubles Du Sommeil, Centre de Recherche CERVO, Institut Universitaire en Santé Mentale de Québec, Canada, and Julie Carrier, Université de Montréal, Hôpital Du Sacré-Cœur de Montréal, Canada, Centre D'étude Avancée en Médecine Du Sommeil, Hôpital Du Sacré-Cœur de Montréal, Canada.

4. Eric Suni & Dr Anis Rehman. Does COVID-19 Cause Sleep Issues Like Insomnia? (sleepfoundation.org) – https://www.sleepfoundation.org/covid-19-and-sleep/covid-insomnia

5. Global prevalence and burden of depressive and anxiety disorders in 204 countries and territories in 2020 due to the COVID-19 pandemic, https://www.thelancet.com/article/S0140-6736(21)02143-7/fulltext

6. The possibility of circadian rhythm disruption in long COVID, https://www.ncbi.nlm.nih.gov/pmc/articles/PMC9153185/

CHAPTER 4

1. Meadows, Dr Guy, *The Sleep Book: How to Sleep Well Every Night* (Orion, 2014)

2. https://knowledge.insead.edu/blog/insead-blog/the-value-lurking-in-your-leadership-unconscious-4974

CHAPTER 5

1. Kets de Vries, M.F.R. & Cheak, A. *Psychodynamic approach* (Faculty & Research Working Paper). (INSEAD, Fontainebleau, 2014). http://sites.insead.edu/facultyresearch/research/doc.cfm?did=54942

CHAPTER 6

1. Sorbonne University, *Napping Reverses Health Effects of Poor Sleep*, Endocrine Society press society, February 10, 2013, www.eurekalert.org

2. Ryan Brindle and Sarah Conklin, *Daytime Sleep Accelerates Cardiovascular Recovery after Psychological Stress*, International Journal of Behavioural Medicine 19 (2012): 111-14

3. *Midday Naps Associated with Reduced Blood Pressure and Fewer Medications*, European Society of Cardiology press release, August 29, 2015, www.escardio.org

4. NASA report by Mark R. Rosekind, Roy M. Smith, Donna L. Miller, Elizabeth L. Co, Kevin B. Gregory, Lissa L. Webbon, Philippa H. Gander & J. Victor Lebacqz, *Alertness Management: Strategic Naps in Operational Settings*, Journal of Sleep Research 4 (1995): 62-66

5. *Neuropsychology: Power Naps Produce a Significant Improvement in Memory Performance*, Science Daily, March 29, 2015, www.sciencedaily.com

6. *Might Lefties and Righties Benefit Differently from a Power Nap?* Georgetown University press release, October 17, 2012, https://explore.georgetown.edu

7. Hideki Tanaka, Kazuhiko Taira, Masashi Arakawa, Hiroki Toguti, Chisae Urasaki, Yukari Yamamoto, Eiko Uezu, Tadao Hori, & Shuichiro Shirakawa, *Effects of Short Nap and Exercise on Elderly People Having Difficulty in Sleeping*, Psychiatry and Clinical Neurosciences 55 (2001): 173-4

8. Sara Mednick, Denise J. Cai, Jennifer Kanady & Sean P.A. Drummond, *Comparing the Benefits of Caffeine, Naps and Placebo on Verbal, Motor and Perceptual Memory*, Behavioural Brain Research 193 (2008): 79-86

CHAPTER 9

1. Compernolle, T., *BrainChains – Discover your brain and unleash its full potential in a hyperconnected multitasking world* (Amsterdam: Compublications, 2014), p.244

2. Matthew Walker, *Why We Sleep* (Penguin 2018), pp.15-17

3. Matthew Walker, *Why We Sleep* (Penguin 2018), p.21

4. Matthew Walker, *Why We Sleep* (Penguin 2018), p.43

5. Lockley, S. W., & Foster, R. G., Sleep: *A very short introduction* (Oxford: Oxford University Press, 2012), pp.56-70

6. Lockley, S. W., & Foster, R. G., Sleep: *A very short introduction* (Oxford: Oxford University Press, 2012), pp.56-70

CHAPTER 10

1. http://healthysleep.med.harvard.edu/healthy/science/what/characteristics

CHAPTER 11

1. https://www.tuck.com/sleep-high

2. http://healthysleep.med.harvard.edu/healthy/science/what/characteristics

3. http://healthysleep.med.harvard.edu/healthy/science/what/characteristics

4. http://healthysleep.med.harvard.edu/healthy/science/what/characteristics

5. http://healthysleep.med.harvard.edu/healthy/science/what/characteristics

6. Matthew Walker, *Why We Sleep* (Penguin 2018), p.207

CHAPTER 12

1. Andrew D. Calvin, Rickey E. Carter, Taro Adachi, Paula G. Macedo, Felipe N. Albuquerque, Christelle van der Walt, Jan Bukartyk, Diane E. Davison, James A. Levine, & Virend K. Somers, *Effects of Experimental Sleep Restriction on Calorie Intake and Activity Energy Expenditure, Chest 144 (2013); 70-86.*

2. Matthew Walker, *Why We Sleep* (Penguin 2018), p.169

3. Lockley, S. W. & Foster, R. G., *Sleep: A very short introduction* (Oxford: Oxford University Press, 2012), pp.79-80

4. Lockley, S. W. & Foster, R. G., *Sleep: A very short introduction* (Oxford: Oxford University Press, 2012), p.84

5. Lockley, S. W. & Foster, R. G., *Sleep: A very short introduction* (Oxford: Oxford University Press, 2012), pp.87-8

CHAPTER 13

1. A.M. Williamson & Anne-Marie Feyer, "Moderate sleep deprivation produces impairments in cognitive and motor performance equivalent to legally prescribed levels of alcohol intoxication," *Occupational and Environmental Medicine*, 2000, Volume 57, Number 10, pp.649-55. Quoted by Nick van Dam and Els van der Helm in "The organizational cost of insufficient sleep," *McKinsey Quarterly* (February 2016)

CHAPTER 15

1. Whitebread, D. & Bingham, S. *Habit formation and learning in young children.* (London, UK: Holborn Centre, 2013). https://financialcapability.gov.au/files/habit-formation-and-learning-in-young-children-uk-2013.pdf

CHAPTER 16

1. Compernolle, T., *BrainChains – Discover your brain and unleash its full potential in a hyperconnected multitasking world* (Amsterdam: Compublications, 2014), p.245

CHAPTER 17

1. Arianna Huffington, *The Sleep Revolution: Transforming Your Life, One Night at a Time* (WH Allen, 2016), pp.20-21

2. Alan Derickson *Dangerously Sleepy*

3. Marie Soderstrom, Kerstin Jeding, Mirjam Ekstedt, Aleksander Perski & Torbjorn Akerstedt, *Insufficient Sleep Predicts Clinical Burnout*, Journal of Occupational Health Psychology 17 (2012): 174-83

4. Kristen L. Knutson, *Sociodemographic and Cultural Determinants of Sleep Deficiency: Implications for Cardiometabolic Disease Risk*, Social Science & Medicine 79 (2013): 7-15.

5. Brian Resnick, *The Black-White Sleep Gap*, National Journal, October 23, 2015, www.nationaljournal.com

CHAPTER 18

1. Arianna Huffington, *The Sleep Revolution: Transforming Your Life, One Night at a Time* (WH Allen, 2016), p.230

2. Charmane I. Eastman & Helen J. Burgess, *How to Travel the World Without Jet Lag*, Sleep Medicine Clinics 4 (2009): 241-55

3. Arianna Huffington, *The Sleep Revolution: Transforming Your Life, One Night at a Time* (WH Allen, 2016), p.233

4. Arianna Huffington, *The Sleep Revolution: Transforming Your Life, One Night at a Time* (WH Allen, 2016), p.234

CHAPTER 19

1. A.Yang, A.A.Palmer & H. de Wit, *Genetics of caffeine consumption and responses to caffeine*, Psychopharmacology 311, no.3 (2010) 245-257 http://www.ncbi.nlm.nih.gov/pmc/articles/PMC4242593/

2. www.scienceDaily.com, June 19, 2012 from the Public Library of Science. Sergio González, David Moreno-Delgado, Estefanía Moreno, Kamil Pérez-Capote, Rafael Franco, Josefa Mallol, Antoni Cortés, Vicent Casadó, Carme Lluís, Jordi Ortiz, Sergi Ferré, Enric Canela & Peter J. McCormick, "Circadian-Related Heteromerization of Adrenergic and Dopamine D4 Receptors Modulates Melatonin Synthesis and Release in the Pineal Gland." *PLoS Biology*, 2012; 10 (6): e1001347 DOI: 10.1371/journal.pbio.1001347)

3. Understanding GABA, *www.thesleepdoctor.com*

4. Yuanyuan Li, Yanil Hao, Fang Fan & Bin Zhang, *"The Role of Microbiome in Insomnia, Circadian Disturbance and Depression,"* The Fronitiers of Psychiatry. (Dec. 2018) retrleved from https://www.ncbi.nlm.nih.gov/pmc/articles/PMC6290721/#!po=0.301205)

5. Matthew Walker, *Why We Sleep* (Penguin, 2018), pp.293-4

6. Rodney K. Dishman, Xuemei Sui, Timothy S. Church, Christopher E. Kline, Shawn D. Youngstedt & Steven N. Blair, *Decline in Cardiorespiratory Fitness and Odds of Incident Sleep Complaints*, Medicine & Science in Sports & Exercise 47 (2015): 960-66

7. *Study: Physical Activity Impacts Overall Quality of Sleep*, Oregon News & Research Communications press release, November 22, 2011, www.oregonstate.edu

8. *Yoga, Running, Weight Lifting, and Gardening: Penn Study Maps the Types of Physical Activity Associated with Better Sleep Habits*, Penn Medicine press release, June 4, 2015, www.uphs.upenn.edu

9. Kelly Glazer Baron, Kathryn J. Reid & Phyllis C. Zee, *Exercise to Improve Sleep in Insomnia: Exploration of the Bidirectional Effects*, Journal of Clinical Sleep Medicine 9 (2013): 819-24

CHAPTER 20

1. Nick van Dam & Els van der Helm, *The organizational cost of insufficient sleep*, McKinsey Quarterly, February 2016

2. Nick van Dam & Els van der Helm, *The organizational cost of insufficient sleep*, McKinsey Quarterly, February 2016

3. Williamson, A. M. & Feyer, A. "Moderate sleep deprivation produces impairments in cognitive and motor performance equivalent to legally prescribed levels of alcohol intoxication." *Occupational and Environmental Medicine, 57* (10), 649-655 (October 2000)

4. Nick van Dam & Els van der Helm, *The organizational cost of insufficient sleep*, McKinsey Quarterly, February 2016

5. *5 areas sleep has the greatest impact on athletic performance*, September 23, 2015, updated May 7, 2019. www.fatiguescience.com

6. Williamson, A. M. & Feyer, A. "Moderate sleep deprivation produces impairments in cognitive and motor performance equivalent to legally prescribed levels of alcohol intoxication." *Occupational and Environmental Medicine, 57* (10), 649-655 (October 2000)

7. Luke A, Lazero RM, Bergeron MF, Keyser L, Benjamin H, Brenner J, d'Hemecourt P, Grady M, Philpott J & Smith A, *Sports-related injuries in youth athletes: is overscheduling a risk factor?* Clinical Journal of Sports Medicine 2011 Jul;21(4): 307-14. Downloaded from ncbi.nlm.nih.gov

8. Winter C. MD, *Studies link fatigue to Major League Baseball (MLB) performance and career longevity*. National Sleep Foundation www.sleepfoundation.org

9. Nick Littlehales, *SLEEP: Redefine Your Rest, for Success in Work, Sport and Life* (Penguin, 2016)

CHAPTER 21

1. Nick van Dam & Els van der Helm, *The organizational cost of insufficient sleep*, McKinsey Quarterly, February 2016.

2. Mohamed Boubekri, Ivy N. Cheung, Kathryn J. Reid, Chia-Hui Wang, & Phyllis C. Zee, *Impact of Windows and Daylight Exposure on Overall Health and Sleep Quality of Office Workers: A Case-Control Pilot Study*, Journal of Clinical Sleep Medicine 10 (2014): 603-11.

3. World Economic Forum LinkedIn Post 23/3/19 (Source: Bloomberg, Footage Crazy Inc.)

4. Arianna Huffington, *The Sleep Revolution: Transforming Your Life, One Night at a Time* (WH Allen, 2016), pp.280-81

CHAPTER 22

1. Meadows, Dr Guy, *The Sleep Book: How to Sleep Well Every Night* (Orion, 2014), p.5

CHAPTER 23

1. Arianna Huffington, *The Sleep Revolution: Transforming Your Life, One Night at a Time* (WH Allen, 2016), p.229

2. Nick Littlehales, *SLEEP: Redefine Your Rest, for Success in Work, Sport and Life* (Penguin, 2016), pp.37-44

3. Magnesium – how it affects sleep. www.thesleepdoctor.com

4. Meadows, Dr Guy, *The Sleep Book: How to Sleep Well Every Night* (Orion, 2014), pp.88-90

5. D.J. Buysse, *Sleep Health: Can we define it? Does it matter?* SLEEP 37, no.1 [2014]: 9-17

CHAPTER 24

1. Extracted from Undergraduate Master's | Centre for Innovation and Entrepreneurship | University of Bristol, 27 February 2024

2. At the time of writing the four-year integrated Master's Innovation Programmes allowed Innovation to be combined with the following: Accounting, Business and Management, Computer Science, Economics, Electrical and Electronic Engineering, Film and Television, Finance, Geography, History, Music, Physics, Psychology and Theatre

3. Extracted from "Challenge: Increasing the Positive Impact of Sleep through Technology" – a Client-led brief for the University of Bristol Centre for Innovation and Entrepreneurship, 2022-3

4. *Team 10 Sleep Well Client Report May 2023* - Lexi Humbert, Freddie Dowland, Gianluca Biancardi, Amy Chappelhow, Michelangelo Khanchandani and Pascha Al-Qassab

5. *Team 3 Report on Technology in Sleep May 2023* - Florence, Jason, Sophia, Martina, Jake, Isobelle

6. *Team 10 Sleep Well Client Report May 2023* - Lexi Humbert, Freddie Dowland, Gianluca Biancardi, Amy Chappelhow, Michelangelo Khanchandani And Pascha Al-Qassab

7. "The experts we interviewed included a university professor of Biomedical Engineering, an Endocrinologist and Nutritionist, a Scientist and President of a neurodegeneration business that implements Red Light Therapy, and a field chiropractor and neurologist." Extracted from *Team 10 Sleep Well Client Report May 2023*

8. "A journey map of their (usual) bedtime routine to help us to understand the motives behind certain actions, as well as any 'pain points' and what is and isn't working well." Extracted from *Team 10 Sleep Well Client Report May 2023*

9. "Cultural probes – research participants were asked (in line with our ethical code of conduct) to take photos of their sleeping environments, sleep technologies, sleep supplements, and wearable sleep aids, in addition to screenshots of apps they've used to aid their sleep. These were revisited as part of the synthesis phase – and helped us get into the real-life problems and to see whether there was disparity between what interviewees were saying to us, and what they were doing in practice." Extracted from *Team 10 Sleep Well Client Report May 2023*

10. Matthew Walker, *Why We Sleep* (Penguin, 2018), extracted from *Team 10 Sleep Well Client Report May 2023*

11. *Team 12 Positive Sleep May 2023* – Jaicheng An, Finn Carter, Issy Chambers, Jessica Pliskin, Sharlotte Santiago and Angus Williams.

12. *Team 12 Positive Sleep May 2023* – Jaicheng An, Finn Carter, Issy Chambers, Jessica Pliskin, Sharlotte Santiago and Angus Williams.